KU-260-493

HEALTH VISITING

PRINCIPLES IN PRACTICE

COUNCIL FOR THE EDUCATION
AND TRAINING OF HEALTH VISITORS

First published in 1982

This book is copyright under the Berne Convention. All rights are reserved. Apart from any fair dealing for the purpose of private study, research, criticism or review, as permitted under the Copyright Act, 1956, no part of this publication may be reproduced, stored in a retrieval system, or transmitted, in any form or by any means, electronic, electrical, chemical, mechanical, optical, photocopying, recording or otherwise, without the prior permission of the copyright owner, to whom enquiries should be addressed.

© Copyright Council for the Education and Training of Health Visitors, 1982.

Published by The Council for the Education and Training of Health Visitors,
Clifton House,
Euston Road,
London.
NW1 2RS

Printed in Great Britain in English Times
by Duncan Printing Co. Limited,
Aylesford, Kent.

Foreword

This document is the third in the series on the principles of health visiting, and expands the work started in "An Investigation into the Principles of Health Visiting" (CETHV 1977) and "The Investigation Debate" (CETHV 1980). Since the last publication appeared a three-day Workshop entitled "Principles in Practice" has been held, which was attended by health visitors representing practitioners, managers and teachers. Some of the papers presented by the speakers at this Workshop, and ensuing discussions, have provided themes which have been developed further in this third book. Other papers have been submitted by interested contributors.

The Council hopes that this document will assist in identifying the ways in which principles can be interpreted in practice, and that it will help to stimulate further discussion and writing on this subject. However these are not definitive statements, and the views expressed are not necessarily those of the Council for the Education and Training of Health Visitors.

In conclusion the Council would like to thank the members of the Working Group on Principles and Practice who have given so much time and consideration to the production of these three publications.

Clifford Butler

Chairman,
Council for the Education and
Training of Health Visitors.

Editorial

This document was edited by the Working Group responsible for the Report 'An Investigation into the Principles of Health Visiting', published CETHV, 1977, and the Report 'The Investigation Debate', published CETHV, 1980.

Membership of the Working Group was -
Miss S.A. Jack (Chairman)
Principal Lecturer in Community Health Studies, Polytechnic of the South Bank.
Miss H.J. Ash
Principal Lecturer in Health Visiting, Gloucestershire College of Arts and Technology.
Miss S.G. Campbell
Principal Lecturer in Health Visiting, Ulster College, The Northern Ireland Polytechnic.
Miss P.R. Hay
Principal Professional Adviser, Council for the Education and Training of Health Visitors
Miss A. Jameson
Professional Adviser, Council for the Education and Training of Health Visitors.
Miss M. McClymont
Principal Lecturer in Health Visiting, Stevenage College of Further Education.
Miss F. Welch
Senior Lecturer in Health Visiting, The Welsh National School of Medicine.
Mrs. M. White
Senior Nursing Officer (Community), Merton, Sutton and Wandsworth Area Health Authority.
Miss H.M. Williams
Principal Lecturer in Health Visiting, Trent Polytechnic, Nottingham
Mrs. C.T. Wilson
Principal Lecturer in Social Policy and Social Administration, North East London Polytechnic.

DISCLAIMER

The views expressed in this publication do not necessarily represent those held either by the employers of the contributors or by the members of the Working Group

Contents

		Page
FOREWORD		3
INTRODUCTION BY CHAIRMAN OF WORKING GROUP — SHEILA JACK		7
CHAPTER 1	SOCIAL SKILL TRAINING FOR HEALTH VISITOR STUDENTS SYLVIA CAMPBELL	10
CHAPTER 2	INTERVENTION IN HEALTH VISITING D. BAHL AND M. McCLYMONT	23
CHAPTER 3	PATHS TO THE VALUE OF HEALTH JUDITH FITTON	28
CHAPTER 4	A SOCIOLOGIST'S VIEW OF HEALTH VISITING SUSAN WILLIS	34
CHAPTER 5	THE DEVELOPMENT OF TEACHING FOR REALITY ALISON McCLYMONT	42
CHAPTER 6	A CASE STUDY IN METHODOLOGY JOB SATISFACTION IN HEALTH VISITING— HOW CAN IT BE MEASURED? PAT ELLIS	55
CHAPTER 7	AN ENQUIRY INTO CHILD HEALTH SURVEILLANCE PROCEDURES UNDERTAKEN BY HEALTH VISITORS IN ENGLAND PHIL CONNOLLY	82
CHAPTER 8	WHAT IS THE HEALTH VISITOR DOING IN EUROPE? THELMA WILSON	100
CHAPTER 9	ABOUT THE ENDS AND MEANS OF HEALTH VISITING RUTH SCHRÖCK	105

Introduction

With the publication of the first two books in this series, 'An Investigation into the Principles of Health Visiting' (CETHV 1977) and 'The Investigation Debate', (CETHV 1980) the Working Group on Principles and Practice (CETHV 1975) began an examination of the value on which health visiting is based and of the consequent principles underlying practice. The subsequent discussion by health visitors and others has underlined the need to continue both theoretical and experimental studies.

Vocational knowledge comprises both theoretical insights and their application. Underlying health visiting is a theory and a body of knowledge about health and its causation, about the identification and assessment of individual, family, and community health, and about the measures and methods that promote health. Traditionally that body of knowledge includes the health of expectant parents and families with young children. The knowledge underlying application is about the relatively more effective promotion of health, for example by:

- using one to one relationships and small peer groups:
- being a service that reaches out to people, working out of the professionals' territory, within people's homes;
- selecting those people who need priority or extra visiting from within apparently homogenous groups;
- using communication techniques (including language) that are apt for the people concerned;
- selecting apt educational methods;
- selecting other methods and techniques apt for promoting health at that time, for that individual, e.g. liaison with other services or referral, observation, examination or screening techniques.

The need is to make explicit the vocational knowledge underlying practice, and thus clarify the relevant attitudes, skills and specific knowledge needed to be able to health visit. One group of health visitors in the Home Counties has been studying practice, but the tools for evaluation still have to be devised. Aspects of this vocational knowledge base and the difficulties in investigating practice are discussed by nine contributors in the following pages. Some of the papers are of a factual nature whilst others pursue new ideas.

Ruth Schröck analyses the work which has been undertaken on principles so far and asserts the need now for empirical investigations into practice by health visitors themselves, so that the knowledge base can be specified more clearly. Susan Willis suggests that sociology can contribute specific knowledge, but more importantly give different perspectives on practice and enhance awareness of the assumptions underlying it. Judith Fitton challenges two perspectives that may limit practice, arguing against the dominance of legitimation by scientific proof alone. In her case study, Pat Ellis discusses one methodology that might be used in empirical investigations.

The analysis of one skill, intervention, by Daman Bahl and Mary McClymont, and the skills-teaching described by Sylvia Campbell focus attention on one aspect of practice, as does Phil Connolly's report of her investigation of another facet, child health surveillance. Preparation for practice by two health visitor courses is examined by Alison McClymont. Thelma Wilson's description of European practice reminds us of the different models possible, and of the imminent requirement to discuss the UK model within the wider framework of the EEC.

The Working Group thanks the authors for their contributions and generous donation of their papers. Individuals have expressed their personal views and the Working Group appreciates the stimulus to thought and knowledge, while not necessarily agreeing with all the points put forward.

It seems timely to express our appreciation of the CETHV's initiation and encouragement of these first attemps to clarify the principles underlying health visitng practice, and therefore education. This kind of creative attitude by a statutory body augers well for any profession, and will be needed within the new statutory education Council and Boards for Nursing, Midwifery and Health Visiting.

Within health visiting, what is needed now are descriptive and analytical studies of practice which are grounded in thorough research methodology and are increasingly undertaken by health visitors. Their publication needs to be not just in the transient form of articles in journals, valuable though these are as a widely available and immediate source of exchange of professional knowledge, but the profession needs to organise publication in permanent form.

Finally, the Working Group thanks all those who have joined in these initial explorations. We have been encouraged by the calibre and potential we have met within our own profession and by the interest and good will of others.

S. Jack

Chapter 1

Social Skill Training for Health Visitor Students

Sylvia Campbell

Health visiting begins at the point of client contact and the essence of effective health visiting lies in the quality of the interaction with the client. From the first encounters with the health visitor, the client will be making a personal judgement of the purpose and usefulness of the service. If the service is perceived by the client as having little relevance for self and/or family and decides not to use it, or perhaps merely to tolerate it, then the aims of health visiting have failed. If on the other hand, the interaction is mutually rewarding, then the health visitor is provided with a firm base from which to proceed with an assessment of the health status of the individual or family from which all further health visiting action and reaction will flow.

As Florence Nightgale wrote in 1891[1] ..."the needs of home health bringing require different qualifications (from that of nursing the sick) ... she (the health visitor) will require tact and judgement unlimited lest the work be regarded as interference and become unpopular." Webster's Dictionary defines tact as "skill or adroitness in doing or saying exactly what is required, a highly developed sense of what is tasteful, proper." Judgement implies power of discrimination, understanding ..."the art or faculty of judging truly, wisely or skillfully, good sense, discernment." In the language of today, tact and judgement may be translated into social skill and it is argued that the possession of highly developed social skills is a pre-requisite for effective health visiting practice.

Orr (1980)[2] in her study of consumer perception of health visiting in Northern Ireland, refers to a degree of discrepancy between what health visitors say they do and what the consumer is aware of them doing. She concludes that the health visitor's social skills appear to be as important as her knowledge base and that consideration should be given to this aspect of training.

The fact that this discrepancy exists can readily be understood when the context of the home visit is considered. It is a relatively simple matter for a health visitor to explain the purpose of a visit, to discuss a child's developmental progress or to carry out a specific procedure such as a screening test for hearing. It is not such a simple matter however for the health visitor to make frequent visits to a family and make explicit that her real concern is about the adequacy of parental care. Where a parent recognises a particular inadequacy in his/her ability to care for a child and seek help, the position is somewhat different. In the former situation, the possession of a range of highly developed social skills or Miss Nightingale's "tact and judgement unlimited" has particular relevance.

How are we to prepare the health visitor student to develop personal awareness and sensitivity to the intangible elements affecting inter-personal relationships; "to develop that skill in establishing inter-personal relationships which will provide a basis for constructive work with families and individuals... to provide practice in working out, with families and individuals, programmes of help where these are required"? (CETHV 1969)[3]

Fortunately, the intangible elements affecting inter-personal relationships are becoming more tangible year by year as the volume of published research evidence continues to grow. Similarly, our access to knowledge of how skills are acquired and developed continues to expand, and advances in educational technology enable us to provide students with an increased range of practice media so that they can rehearse their skills in a variety of controlled environments where they can receive audio-visual feedback on their performance before, and at intervals during, their professional career.

However, it is one thing to have an accumulated body of knowledge and the means to transmit the knowledge, it is quite another problem to integrate various forms of knowledge and relate this to practice. The dilemmas surrounding the integration of theory and practice of health visiting led to the beginning of the current investigation into the principles of health visiting.[4]

In addressing the problems raised by the injunction to relate theory and practice, Ellis and Whittington (1981)[5] provide a helpful analysis of this apparently universally difficult problem. Their analysis relates to the provision of courses of education and training for what they term "the interpersonal professions". These professions are defined as those which rely on dyadic or small group interaction as their prime means of achievement of their objectives. The professions considered span the education, health and personal social services and include health visitor education and training.

In their analysis, the authors conceive theoretical propositions relating to professional action to exist at least three levels and they label these levels of theory as follows:

"(1) PERSONAL THEORY: the implicit and occasionally explicit set of assumptions regarding purpose and practice which the student brings to the course.

(2) PROFESSIONAL THEORY: the explicit theory associated with professional practice and expounded by professional tutors and supervisors.

(3) ACADEMIC THEORY: the set of propositions contributed by academic disciplines deemed for various reasons to be relevant to to the profession concerned."

Applying this analysis to health visiting, it can be said that health visitors and health visitor students will bring to their practice, their own views, assumptions and values regarding health visiting interaction. It is likely that these students in particular will be strongly influenced by their previous nursing and midwifery or obstetric experience. The latter experience could be regarded as the transition from the illness/pathology orientation of nursing to the health visitor point of entry, which is contact with the well population, typically the family with the new baby, but many students will not have accommodated this conceptual shift. For other students their assumptions about health visiting interaction will have been influenced by experience as consumers of the service.

In relation to professional theory, the students will be exposed to the body of knowledge and values held by tutors, fieldwork teachers, supervisors, managers and other health visitors, as well as from the professional literature. (See for example Dingwall (1977)[6] and Ellis P.[7])

In terms of academic theory they will be exposed to knowledge, models and standards of evidence regarding interpersonal interaction from a range of sources including psychology, social psychology and sociology.

These three levels of theory require to be integrated with health visiting practice. At this stage of the analysis, the authors introduce a further complication; the distinction between descriptive and prescriptive forms of theory. They remind us that the academic disciplines are by definition descriptive only, whereas professional theory must be prescriptive, otherwise it fails in its job. While personal theory can operate at descriptive and prescriptive levels, and to some extent, professional theory also, academic theory should be descriptive only, on principle. The complexity of this matrix of levels of theory in prescriptive and descriptive forms is, they suggest, the basis of much contention within course teams wrestling with the injunction to plan courses which demonstrate the relationship between theory and practice. As Ruth Schröck[8] points out, there is no way in which psychology or sociology can explain health visiting in health visiting terms; they can explain it in psychological or sociological terms, and it is only health visitors who can explain health visiting in health visiting terms.

Ellis and Whittington go on to describe what they term an "Action Focus" curriculum model, exemplified by social skill training, which they propose as the most thoroughly worked out example of a curriculum unit which makes professional action its focus. (For further elaboration of this model see "The Curriculum Context" in Ellis and Whittington 1981[9])

Briefly, the model they propose necessitates "close analysis of professional practice and skills including interpersonal skills. Learning experiences are then devised so that a student can integrate his developing capacity to articulate and comprehend propositions with his selection, implementation and evaluation of various courses of professional action".

The case study which follows is a descriptive account of a social skill training programme for health visitor students which attempts to follow the "Action Focus" model described above.

Social Skill training for Health Visitor Students - A Case Study

History of the emergence and development of the Social Skill Training Programme (SST)

When the health visitor training course which had been established in Northern Ireland since 1948 transferred to the Ulster Polytechnic in 1972, a new and extended range of teaching and learning resources were opened up. This was due partly to the centralisation of staffing resources which brought together staff from a wide range of academic, professional and technical areas all with their own particular expertise, and partly to developments in educational technology.

One of those resources which has since proved to be of major importance in the area of professional skill training for a wide range of courses within the Polytechnic was the SST Unit where microteaching had been established for teacher training programmes.

The health visitor course tutor at that time, together with the staff from contributing disciplines recognised the potential of this training method for health visitor students. It had originally been envisaged mainly as a preparation for the students' future group teaching activities in the area of health education. Further discussions between the staff involved led to the decision to adopt the microteaching programme to focus on the skills of interviewing, counselling and teaching in the dyadic situation, as well as some group teaching skills. This process became known as micro-counselling.

After an appropriate period of training for the staff to be involved, a programme of training was introduced for our first intake of students who were then midway through their course.

The skills initially chosen for analysis and practice were:

set induction (opening the visit/interview/teaching session);

use of questions;

reinforcement of client/interviewee/pupil responses (verbal and non-verbal);

stimulus variation;

explaining;

demonstrating;

closure (closing the visit/interview/teaching session);

integration of skills.

During the course of our nine years experience, this basic programme has been extended, modified and refined in the light of further research findings in the area of social skill training, feedback from students at the end of the course, feedback from former students who are now established practitioners, and feedback from the tutors involved.

These additions, modifications and refinements have included:

(1) changes in the timing of the training programme which is now introduced during the first week of the course and continues for the first half of the academic year;

(2) changes in the sequence of skills analysed and practised in order to achieve better integration with other aspects of the course, particularly fieldwork practice;

(3) the inclusion of additional skills i.e. non-verbal communication, reflection of feeling and sustaining, and group discussion skills with particular emphasis on leadership tasks and styles;

(4) increased emphasis on the familiarisation phase to create a more relaxed learning environment and allow students time to adjust to the cosmetic effect of seeing and hearing themselves;

(5) change in description of the process from "microcounselling" to "social skill training".

The course team have adopted the definition derived by Hargie et al (1981)[10] that social skill is "a set of goal-directed, interrelated social behaviours which can be learned and which are under the control of the individual."

A stated aim of the health visiting course is "that students will develop interpersonal skills which will form a basis for constructive work with families and individuals." In relation to this broad aim, the social skill training component of the course has been designed with the following specific aims:

(1) to encourage a sense of critical awareness of self and others in social situations;

(2) to facilitate the identification, analysis, discrimination and practice of specified social skills;

(3) to relate the study of social skills to the professional context of health visiting; and

(4) to relate the practical application of social skills to a theoretical framework derived from the social psychology of group and dyadic interaction.

Description of Present Procedures

1. Introduction and Familiarisation.

This includes discussion of the SST programme in relation to the course objectives, the rationale of SST as a teaching method, and introduction to the SST centre and its layout, equipment and resources.

Students are given detailed timetables of the practical activities to be undertaken each week, and of the associated lectures and demonstrations. They also receive guidelines on the preparatory reading and follow-up activities required. More detailed guidance is given from week to week as the course progresses. This takes place in the theoretical classes which precede each practice session.

In our experience, the careful planning and management of this phase in order to allay anxiety and create a pleasant and relaxed learning environment is crucial to the success of the entire programme.

2.   Logistics.

   (1) Students work in groups (ideally 6 in each group) with a tutor.
   (2) Each group is allocated to one of the training units which comprises a suite of two adjacent rooms. One room contains all the equipment necessary for videotaping and viewing student performance. The second room is where the students undertake their practice sessions. It is simply furnished with a range of easily movable chairs and tables of various kinds. Students can arrange the furniture to experiment with various seating arrangements and simulate the desired setting e.g. home, clinic, office or classroom. The TV camera and microphone are positioned inconspicuously at ceiling level.
   (3) Each student role plays with a colleague or colleagues from the group in a health visiting situation specified by the tutor. The situations are chosen to allow opportunity for practice of the skill under consideration. This interaction is recorded on videotape.
   (4) When each student has participated in the role of health visitor and of client, all students in the group come together with their tutor to the first room to view and analyse the interaction.
   (5) The videotapes are then erased for subsequent re-use. No taped material is used for demonstration purposes to other groups without prior permission from the students concerned.

3.   Follow-up.

It has been found to be beneficial for students to keep a written record of their experience as the course progresses. This may take the form of a log-book where students record their own progress from week to week and enter examples of how they were able to use particular skills during fieldwork practice which takes place concurrently.

Typically, such a log-book would contain:
1. (1) an analysis of the rationale for SST;
2. (2) a summary of each of the social skills studied together with anticipated implications for professional interaction;
3. (3) an evaluation of these skills in the light of experience in the SST Unit, in the Polytechnic generally, and in fieldwork practice;
4. (4) a summative evaluation of SST work and experience;
5. (5) any innovatory ideas which have occured to the student e.g. a social skill not included in the programme which may be important in health visiting practice.

Alternatively, students may be asked at intervals during the course, to undertake short written assignments incorporating the elements itemised in (1) - (5) above.

Students are encouraged to discuss the content of their log-book or written assignments with their fieldwork teachers, and the material provided forms the basis of individual tutorials where individual strengths and weaknesses can be identified and further guidance provided as appropriate.

The Place of Social Skill Training in the Curriculum

The health visiting course is one of more than twenty professional courses within the Faculty of Social and Health Sciences. While most of these courses are subject to external validation by the appropriate professional body, they are all subject to internal validation at faculty and institutional level.

Reference has already been made to the benefits of sharing experiences and resources within a polytechnic setting. This is particularly true in relation to the internal course validation processes which have facilitated the identification of common themes and common concerns across a wide range of professional courses. In this context, the integration of theory and practice can be seen to be a universally challenging concern and one that is not in any way peculiar to health visiting. It can also be seen that ways of resolving the dilemmas surrounding the integration of theory and practice can most readily be found when experience is shared within and between course teams.

Commenting on the advantages for the profession of the location of courses for education and training of health visitors within higher education settings, Batley (1980)[11] points out that "nothing would be more deadening to the service than the complacent continuation of the same practices year after year." She refers to the bridging of theory and practice which is facilitated when professional tutors and academic theorists are in a working situation where they can "sharpen their wits on each other" in critical yet constructive manner.

Arising from the multidisciplinary and multiprofessional membership of course teams working together within this Faculty, a model for curriculum development for professional courses has been developed which is described as an "Action Focus" model.[12]

In this model, the curriculum is focused on the acquisition of professional skills and knowledge directly related to these skills (competency based study); and knowledge which provides a context for the operation of the skills (contextual studies). This distinction between competency based and contextual studies has been a useful frame of reference for the course team in devising a programme of polytechnic based and field based experiences to facilitate the development of health visiting skills.

It has been argued earlier that the possession of highly developed social skills is a pre-requisite for effective and client-centred visiting practice. The aims of the social skill training programme have also been stated in relation to one of the major course aims concerned with the development of interpersonal skills. Social skill training therefore is allocated a central place in the curriculum for the first half of the course and 90 curriculum hours are devoted to SST theory and practice in the ratio 2:4.

The competency based study is the theory from psychology and social psychology which is directly related to the skill under consideration, and the contextual study takes place in other elements of the course e.g. principles and practice of health visiting (polytechnic and field-based), psychology, sociology, social aspects of health and disease and social policy.

Comparison of Social Skill Training with Previous Procedures with similar aims.

Before the introduction of SST the training methods used locally included lecture, discussion, direct observation by the student of practising health visitors, and direct observation of the student by the tutor. The use of role play, audiotape and film had been developed to some extent. SST combines the best features of the previous methods, and has additional advantages. The most outstanding advantage is the availability of instant feedback on verbal and non-verbal performance. The videotape can be stopped at any point for analysis of a particular episode in the interaction and can be rewound and replayed as often as required. The students response to verbal and non-verbal cues is immediately obvious and a whole previously hidden area of behaviour is revealed to the person concerned. The student experiences what it is like to be at both the giving and receiving end of the interview, visit or lesson; experience for him/herself the effects of different levels of questioning; can appreciate the irritating effect of advice being dispensed before efforts are made to establish the present state of the patient's/client's knowledge or can appreciate the ineffectiveness or potentially dangerous effects of badly structured and incomplete explanations of the management of particular health problems. In short, the student can see for himself how easily home visits or clinic consultations can so easily become ritualised performances of no real value to any of the participants.

The student is enabled to experiment with a range of interviewing/counselling/teaching styles and techniques in a variety of simulated settings in the safe environment of the classroom before encountering the real situation. Not only is the student enabled to see his own performance, but he/she can see how colleagues perform in a similar situation. These tapes can then be compared with the demonstration tapes and the student has a model at which to aim.

Another advantage of SST over previous methods lies in its flexibility. The pace and sequence of the programme can be controlled by the tutors in order to best meet the objectives of the training programme. The tutor has available a taped profile of each student and can identify individual strengths and weaknesses. Because the students work in small groups with a tutor, the danger of missing some students in difficulty is minimised.

The content of the interactions can also be examined as well as the process, although care must be taken discussion of content does not divert attention from the skill analysis which is the main focus of the programme.

Student and Staff Attitudes to SST

Students.

It is not unusual for a number of students to approach this part of the course with some degree of trepidation. This can range from a mixture of self consciousness and excited curiosity to real anxiety about role playing and being televised. Such attitudes are manifested in a range of behaviours from self conscious giggles and whispers to open hostility. "Do we really have to do this?" is a question which has been asked from time to time.

Another attitude which has been noted could be described as: "The don't teach your granny to suck eggs" syndrome. This is the view that anyone who has nursing and midwifery experience has nothing more to learn about social skill.

Other students appear enthusiastic and confident at the beginning but can experience a "let down" later on when they find themselves unable to achieve a desired performance after a series of successful ones. This can be likened to the process of acquiring complex motor skills e.g. learning to drive or play golf, when performance does not progress in a uniform way (Argyle 1972)[13], and demonstrates the importance of the familiarisation phase and the linked theory. Only as the students' understanding of the communication process itself increases, as their self awareness and sensitivity to others increases, do these attitudes modify and for some students this takes a considerable time.

A current research project is concerned with evaluation of the SST programme for health visitor students in relation to individual differences which may be affecting achievement.

Staff Attitudes.

College Staff.

In the earlier years of our venture into the realms of SST, recollections and impressions of staff attitudes are that they contained varied ingredients of enthusiasm, conviction, apprehension and caution with a pinch of scepticism.

There was some concern about the time factor involved from a staff and student perspective. The course was already considered to be heavily timetabled and at this stage there was insufficient confidence in our knowledge about SST upon which to base decisions about reducing the time given to other areas of the course. This kind of problem will always confront any course committee operating within their own particular resource constraints and within the requirements of the particular course validating body.

Some of the caution, apprehension and scepticism was related to the technical aspects: our own lack of confidence in our ability to control the equipment; the fallibility of machines and power supplies and the logistics of the whole procedure. These reservations were overcome to a great extent by a staff training programme where we practised with each other and learned how to improvise when technical hitches did occur.

This staff training programme also helped us to resolve the concern which had been expressed as to possible traumatic side effects on students. We learned that the programme accommodated an inbuilt counselling system and that in fact many of our expressions of concern contained an element of rationalisation of our own lack of experience in this field. It is likely also that some of these attitudes were compounded by the fact that we were also in the process of establishing ourselves in a new environment. This kind of reservation is not now apparent in the attitude of more recently qualified tutors who have experienced micro teaching in their own training courses.

Field Staff.

At every stage of the development of the programme efforts were made to keep field staff informed of the polytechnic based aspects of training. This was achieved by formal and informal discussions with staff at all levels and in particular the fieldwork teachers who form the most vital link between the polytechnic and the field. It is the fieldwork teacher who is the first and most influential role model for the student, and who must be informed and in accord with current training procedures if the programme is to be fully effective.

The geographical location of Northern Ireland results in a relatively stable population of health visitors, and a stage has now been reached when the majority of entrants to the fieldwork teachers' course which is now provided in the Polytechnic, will have experienced social skill training in their own health visitor training course.

The student subsequently is influenced by a widening range of field staff, and his/her competence is finally assessed by a Nursing Officer.

Until we reach a stage when we have developed a common language for the description of professional skills which can be shared by Polytechnic staff, field staff and students we will continue to be beset by problems of reliability and validity in the assessment of practical competence.

This ideal model of a common language for the description of professional skills has implications for (a) education of college staff (b) education of students and (c) education of fieldworkers.

References

1. Selected Writings of Florence Nightingale 1981. Quoted in McEwan M. *Health Visiting.* Faber and Faber. London 1952. (Second Edition p.20.)
2. Orr J.A. *Health Visiting in Focus.* RCN. London 1980.
3. Council for the Education and Training of Health Visitors. Fourth Report 1969.
4. Working Group Report *An Investigation into the principles of Health Visiting.* CETHV. London 1977. p.7.
5. Ellis R. and Whittington D. *A Guide to Social Skill Training.* Croom Helm. London 1981. (Chap. 6 "The Curriculum Context" pages 162-166)
6. Dingwall R. *The Social Organisation of Health Visitor Training* Croom Helm. London 1977. (Chap. 3 "Theories of Society")
7. See Chap. 6. Ellis P. *A Case Study Methodology*
8. See Chap. 9. Schöck R. *About the Ethics and Means of Health Visiting*
9. Ellis R. and Whittington D. Ibid. Pages 171-177.
10. Hargic O., Saunders C. and Dickson D. *Social Skills in Interpersonal Communication.* Croom Helm. London 1981. (pages 13-14)
11. Batley N. *Education and Training for Primary Care as seen by a Health Visitor.* Nursing Times Occasional Papers Vol 76. No. 10. 1980.
12. Ellis R. and Whittington D. Ibid. Pages 171-177.
13. Argyle M. *The Psychology of Interpersonal Behaviour.* Penguin Hammondsworth 1972. (Chap. 3 "Social Skill")

Chapter 2

Intervention in Health Visiting

Daman Bahl and Mary McClymont

Health visitors require to have access to a wide range of skills: of these skills an important one is intervening. Intervention has many connotations, not all of which are acceptable to health visitors. The dictionary[1] states that intervention is 'coming between'. Where intervention is action taken positively with individuals, groups or communities it is acceptable to health visitors but where it can be perceived as interference, it is not. The following definition, arrived at during the Brighton Workshop,* appears to be helpful 'to intervene as a health visitor is to enter into a continuing system of relationships, to come between or among persons or groups for the purpose of helping towards positive health'. Health promotion measures are interventions in life events and crises.

In considering the ethics of intervention, health visitors often ask such questions as 'can we actually intervene?', 'are we justified in intervening?', 'do we have the right to intervene?', Yet even a health visitor conversing with a client is a form of intervention since the person is diverted from whatever they might originally have been doing. This may appear obvious, but a closer examination of this process will be helpful.

Murray and Zentner[2] state that all actions that you carry out to promote the patient's/client's adaption comprise intervention, the third step in the nursing process. You intervene (from the latin meaning come between) when you modify, settle or hinder some action in order to prevent harm or further dysfunction.

A health visiting intervention has occured whether or not an action is modified in order to prevent harm or further dysfunction. The qualifying element therefore lies in the motive for which the intervention is

* Many of the ideas contained in this chapter derive from the CETHV Workshop, Principles in Practice, Brighton 1981.

23

undertaken, otherwise the action could be construed as malicious or interfering. Thus it can be seen that health visiting intervention must not be undertaken lightly or precipitately, for although intervention may be undertaken with best intentions, adaptation may not occur. Health visitors must constantly remind themselves that it is the client who makes the adaptation. One interpretation of intervention is planning and creating an environment appropriate to the whole person. It includes the empathetic offering of self for strength to clients when they are bewildered, confused or distressed; the counselling and teaching of clients when they require the clarification of issues, feel the need to talk out problems or require specific and accurate information on health matters. It includes interactive discussion and exploration of thoughts and feelings so that adaptive and adequate responses can be made by the individual client and by client groups. Intervention includes the proper use of the social and political systems to create an environment conducive to health.

Intervention may be regarded as a continuum in health visiting practice. On analysis, it seems that intervention represents the application of the four principles of health visiting[3] in practice. This can be seen, first, when examining the search principle, for example, in carrying out the search for health needs, the health visitor may intervene by contacting various services in an area in order to identify patterns of health and disease, population structure and other factors determining the health states and needs of the inhabitants.

Second, the ways in which health visitors may attempt the stimulation of the awareness of health needs may involve health education for individuals resulting eventually in a greater awareness in the community of its specific needs.

Third, the influencing of policies affecting health obviously necessitates intervention in terms of altering the status quo. Increasingly, health visitors are aware of the opportunities open to them to work at multidisciplinary, national and international levels. Communication, political and social skills with the relevent knowledge are therefore vital to the health visitor. This same health visitor will raise the question as to who has the responsibility for the health state of the people in general, and in the area in which she works in particular.

Fourth, similarly in organising the facilitation of health enhancing activities, intervention is involved because the health visitor is encouraging clients to think in a particular way in order to make it easier for the client to use the services which are available.

The conclusion to be drawn from this brief analysis is that intervention is inherent in health visiting. The questions to be examined do not, therefore, focus on whether one should intervene but rather, on how one should intervene, on the degree and type of intervention.

Some interventions, such as, comfort measures and hygiene instruction, are clear cut situations; planning and creating a healthy environment, which includes health teaching and protection from risk of injury, fits the health visiting credo. Other forms of intervention may be more problematic and in considering when and how health visitors should intervene, the six category analysis of Heron et al.[4] provides a helpful framework;

1. **prescriptive intervention:** directing the client's attention to behaviour beyond the interaction (anticipatory guidance). It may refer to current or future behaviour and the client is free to accept/reject,
2. **informative intervention:** the giving of knowledge or information to the client relevant to need,
3. **confronting intervention:** the challenging of attitudes or behaviour of the client, whilst at the same time giving support,
4. **cathartic intervention:** encouraging client to laugh/cry etc. as providing a reaction for some painful emotion, but done at a level with which the clients can cope,
5. **catalytic intervention:** encouraging self-direction and self-discovery by the client within interactive relationships,
6. **supportive intervention:** caring, genuine and intimate, showing the work of the client and the worker or counsellor's approval of the client.

Prescriptive intervention, often called anticipatory guidance, is an important aspect of routine health visiting. Although health visitors are not involved in clinical therapeutic relationships, the long term nature of their contact places great responsibility on them for planned prescriptive intervention. For this to be effective local and national epidemiological and statistical information needs to be made readily available. At the same time, personal health, social and cultural data should be shared by professional colleagues, within the limits of confidentiality.

Informative intervention, though a part of routine health visiting, is shaped and personalised to meet each client's unique need. Intervention has many connotations ranging from unsolicited advice to consultancy. To achieve health visiting intervention, more awareness of self and of personal preferences is needed on the part of both client and health visitor. Such personal revelation may come about not only through understanding social psychology but also philosophy.

Thus the basis of trust between the health visitor and client depends on their mutual understanding. There needs to be awareness of emotions, reactions, heightened sensitivities and acceptance of social and cultural differences.

Health visitors have been traditionally involved in health education which may require 'confronting' intervention techniques. Clients who smoke, over-eat, over indulge in alcohol, may resent being presented with information by the health visitor, whereas health visitors consider that, in this situation, they are acting for the client's good.

A rather less frequently used skill of health visiting is that of cathartic intervention. This is perhaps most frequently used in bereavement counselling.

Of all forms of health visiting intervention that of catalytic intervention is perhaps the most basic as it relates to every encounter with individuals, groups or communities.

Increasingly, health visitors seem to be involved in more work of supportive intervention, but traditionally they have intervened supportively at critical points in the life cycle, often in an unobtrusive way. Some aspects of this intervention have to be immediate. This is a confusing term since it applies to the situation rather than the type of intervention.

Where appropriate, health visitors will intervene in a group or, alternatively, a number of health visitors may work together with a group of people where they have a common focus. This type of intervention will require different awareness and skill but it is equally as valuable to the community as the work that is done with families.

A generic approach to health visiting is often used in explaining the ideal role, yet, because of staff shortages and 'priority setting', the generic model is rarely implemented in practice. The availability and accessibility of health visitors is closely linked with the development of health visiting intervention.

Intervention in health visiting can further be characterized by the three stages noted by Argyris[5] when discussing general intervention theory and method:

1. the generation of valid information.
2. the maintenance of client autonomy and free, informed choice, and

3. the on-going maintenance of client autonomy using all available systems, so that the commitment of the client to learning and change is more or less permanent and can be transferred.

The importance of the need for valid, or accurate, information is high-lighted in the light of clients' perceptions of the health visitor. They expect her to be an expert in health matters. Obviously the need for ongoing education, research and documentation of health visiting practice is necessary. For the health visiting intervention to be credible there must be accurate information to offer clients and such can only be obtained through research. There is not an immutable and unchanging body of knowledge. New information has to be validated before it can be accepted.

Health visitors must be sure that they are not tossed about by every new theory, and that they examine each in the light of current knowledge and experience, so that the intervening action is based on a sound rationale. External constraints may affect the use of data, whilst shortage of time, large case loads and employer's dictates may affect and even prevent the possibility of health visitors themselves undertaking research and thus making a contribution to the development of the knowledge base. This is important if one considers whence health visitors derive their knowledge.

Health visiting would seem to be eclectic in that it uses knowledge derived from a variety of supporting disciplines as diverse as genetics and microbiology on the one hand and moral philosophy and economics on the other. Each discipline can add something to health visiting, but it is the extrapolation of the relevant which is crucial to the further development of the theoretical base of health visiting.

Finally, if health visiting is interventionist action aimed at adaptation for health and development, then it is a valuable, dynamic and interactive process which should be available throughout all strata of society and all age groups.

References

1. Oxford English Dictionary
2. Murray R B and Zentner JP *Nursing Concepts for Health Promotion* Prentice Hall inc. New Jersey. (1979) p. 121.
3. CETHV *An Investigation into the Priniciples of Health Visiting* (1977) p.9
4. Heron J *Six Category Intervention Analysis* University of Surrey (1975)
5. Argyris C *Intervention Theory and Method: A Behaviourial Science View* Addison Wesley (1970) p.17.

Chapter 3

Paths to the Value of Health

Judith M. Fitton

It is ironical, but quite natural, that even while we discuss the nature of health visiting practice, that practice and the balance of values on which it is based are changing around us. There is a strong and persuasive factor at large in today's primary health care teams which at this time has a reducing effect on the scope and quality of health visiting practice. This factor is the pressure to reduce health visiting practice to the known scientific. Some, who hold materialist values of hard science will say it is for the better, while others, acknowledging wider values, will say it is for the worse.

Health visitors put effort into trying, as human to human, to influence their clients to live and act in ways deemed beneficial to themselves, their families, and society. When health visitors descibe to co-workers in the health field their work with clients, some self-valued bits of what they do can be challenged as being "non-scientific". Some can be challenged by an observer as being of little practical significance when seen against that observer's values. An example of this might be the judgement passed upon an effort to motivate an elderly person consciously to adopt a diet containing vitamin C. The challenge to this health visiting activity might suggest that it is of little value in the absence of any clinical evidence of scurvy. Such challenges ocurring amongst primary health care team members constitute the agenda out of which the team builds its shared and agreed values. Who conforms with whom? What is the orthodoxy of belief in a health care team consisting of general practitioners, nurses and health visitors?

The health visiting perspective of work with clients is different from the mainstream general nursing perspective (before V. Henderson[1], and the 1979 Panel of Assessors Curriculum in district Nursing for State Registered Nurses and Registered General Nurses[2], I hasten to add) in that the 'mainstream-general' has been bound in the manner of a three-legged race to the perspective held by the medical profession. By the 'perspective' of these professions is meant the assumptions, being values and beliefs, which members of the profession take for granted that they share with each other, and which underlie their practice. In this context, then, the assumptions underlying the practice of health visiting hinge primarily on the value ascribable to the condition of mankind known as 'health', and the belief that the repertoire of health visiting activities has the potential for developing 'health' in the client population. The principles which identify and guide health visiting practice stem from these assumptions. A health visiting theory seems to be grounded in the repertoire of activities available to health visitors, according to the principles and values of the profession, in and with regard to the client's own environment and milieu.

Essentially, each client's milieu is unique, being composed of an infinity of historical, genetic, physical, environmental, and social-dependency variables. Health visiting theory takes cognisance of those variables. I anticipate that at this point some readers will be happy to agree that health visitors at large do indeed value the individuality and even the perversity of humanity. On health matters and from experience, clients are only rational if you can persuade them to be so, and if they have knowledge enough to think rationally through the alternatives when they make their choices. Other readers will find agreement uncomfortable and these are the adherents to 'scientific method' as the sole criterion of value in health promotion.

Approval by primary health care team colleagues is most likely to be given to those visiting activities which are based on 'scientific method'. An unwary visitor may get caught in the 'reinforcement' web by virtue of 'learning' from such selective approval and thus increase his or her output of these specific activities, whilst he or she justifies the change on the grounds of shared values. Screening activities are such examples. Already we see some health visiting practices built exclusively round birth dates and screening programmes.

Consider though - this 'scientific method' has a modern scientific materialism as its 'taken for granted' virtue and value.

Scientific laws, 'science' itself, and scientific method have in the past been thought to exist in nature independent of man. More recently it has been recognised that they are in fact highly dependent on man since man in the capacity of observer or experimenter, always distorts that which is studied. Scientific method is thus always 'subjective' to a greater or lesser degree. Similarly, the entities to be studied vary in the degree in which they lend themselves to predictability and scientific method. In physics, for instance, scientific laws have always proved to be eminently discoverable by man, and it is possible to predict within the conditions of known law. In biology on the other hand this cannot take place, as man's understanding of events is too primitive. Medical practice therefore has in the past had recourse largely to the use of the laws of physics to solve the problems of human biology.

Rhodes in his book 'The Value of Medicine'[3] from which some of these ideas are derived, writing of conditions in the 18th Century, sees in "Newtonian Medicine" practice in which the patient is passive as he presents himself to the doctor "very much like a lump of matter without antecedents and without potential. He was here and now, and treated in isolation from his surrounding just as scientists thought they could investigate matter. The unacknowledged code of materialism reigned in the practice of medicine."

Rhodes[4] goes on to say that this materialism has not been fully modified at the present time. He wonders if sociology will enable a new framework to be devised for medical and health care practice?

In the meantime, what of these health care activities which do not follow predictable outcomes? Who of us as health visitors will insist, against pressure, that we prize informal health teaching with client X in his/her home, as much as the screening of Baby Y or of diabetic patient Z?

Where the pressures are on the health visitor to bias his or her work in the direction of activities having clear and acknowledged scientific method, it is likely that preference will also be given to those activities which take place in an environment which allows controls of the obvious variables (for example the surgery, clinic or classroom). Both of these in turn constrain the catholicity of a 'theory' of health visiting and potentially eliminate its uniqueness in the "search for health needs". In addition these constraints have the potential of medicalizing health needs which would not otherwise be seen as either illness or sickness related. Rhodes claims that the specialist health care groups (which, he says, have "spawned" themselves in the community,) serve to "reproduce and generate ill-health by raising expectations and definitions".[5] This claim can be refuted by the health visiting profession which, to the contrary, spawns workers who lead the health care field in defining people as clients, and thus autonomous, rather than as patients and thus dependent.

"For various reasons it is difficult to apply the scientific method in full to human beings ... It is suggested that there is another dimension in addition to the scientific in the health visitor's methods .." (Investigation into the Principles of Health Visiting[6]). Campbell in his book "Medicine Health and Justice"[7] deduces from Kant's philosophy that "systems which take away autonomy treat people partially or reduce individuals to the status of things cannot be regarded as genuinely moral systems". The author goes on to suggest that in medical practice "priority should be given to those medical interventions most likely to increase autonomy amongst those least able to exercise it without outside help." He then names the priorities as children in deprived areas, the elderly and the mentally handicapped. "All these are on the outer fringes of scientific medicine. The skills they demand are more in the realm of relationships than in the sphere of biological research and physical treatment."[8]

Riding in tandem with the high value attached to activities visibly using scientific method is the value attached to activities which are demonstrably successful in cost effectiveness terms. Health visitors themselves rarely innovate such activities and the notion of the 'commercial element' in health care tends to stem from the political and resource planning strategies of the governing authorities. These same sources in the governing authorities have, however, been known to switch the notion of a fiscal valuation attached to some health care activities into the mechanistic proposition that all health care activities 'should' be measurable in cost-benefit terms. This idea stems from the precocious belief that since cosmic order pervades, it must be specifiable and demonstrable in the microcosmic affairs of men within the governed organisation. Health visitors may well join with social workers in saying that the possibility of achieving such measurement for more than a small proportion of their activities is in inverse ratio to the variables which impinge on their clients. Managers, health care policy makers and planners with insights into the wider and more educational view of the contribution of health visiting in the health care services may possibly find themselves beset by the same materialistic pressures from other 'team members' as potentially beset the health visitor. Health visiting can easily live with a multiple value system, incorporating both scientific method (materialistic values) and a pragmatic method (holistic values) - with both the medical and educational models - but holding to the dichotomy cannot be easy for individual workers if the same range of values does not occur elsewhere amongst the team members.

The future may well be moving in the direction of recognition of the 'humanist' values in medical and nursing practice.

Research which gives 'scientific' knowledge of man, his health and his social behaviour is, at the present time, incredibly rudimentary. Certainly

**Diagram showing the value orientations
of health visiting practice.**

The dichotomy
of values

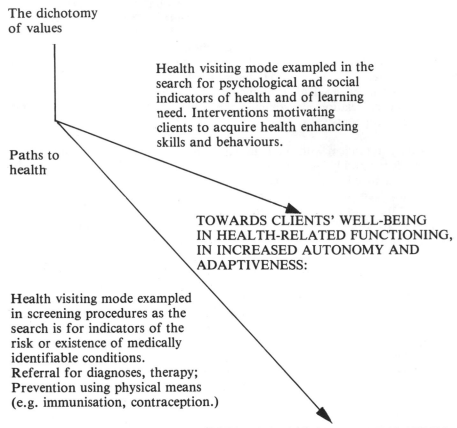

Health visiting mode exampled in the
search for psychological and social
indicators of health and of learning
need. Interventions motivating
clients to acquire health enhancing
skills and behaviours.

Paths to
health

TOWARDS CLIENTS' WELL-BEING
IN HEALTH-RELATED FUNCTIONING,
IN INCREASED AUTONOMY AND
ADAPTIVENESS:

Health visiting mode exampled
in screening procedures as the
search is for indicators of the
risk or existence of medically
identifiable conditions.
Referral for diagnoses, therapy;
Prevention using physical means
(e.g. immunisation, contraception.)

TOWARDS THE CURE, MITIGATION
OR AVOIDANCE OF MEDICALLY
IDENTIFIABLE CONDITIONS OF
THE PATIENT.

health care workers should know of and make appropriate use of the
knowledge which exists. At the same time we should recognise the
limitations of this knowledge. Vast unknowns also exist and day by day we
live with these, dealing with them in everyman's relationship with
everyman, by guess and by custom, by perception of right, of truth and
beauty and of the desirable and the undesirable. Doctors deal with these

unknowns by guess and by custom - and by the rest; so do scientists and so do health visitors in their practice. Custom serves the essential purpose of enabling the social continuity of the species, its coping and adaptation, in a word, its mental health.

Virginia Henderson[9] includes in her description of basic nursing care the activity of enabling the patient to "learn, discover, or satisfy the curiosity that leads to normal development and health and use the available health facilities." This activity is emminently identifiable as a core health visiting function, but it is equally desirable as a mainstream nursing function, and indeed, as a function of all other health care workers. If the future brings more educational skill and awareness to those who work in the primary health care team alongside health visitors, it is all to the good. Perhaps then the balance of values in ways and means on the path to health will achieve equilibrium.

References

1. Henderson, Virginia *The Nature of Nursing* The Macmillan Company 1966
2. Panel of Assessors for District Nurse Training *Curriculum in District Nursing for State Registered Nurses and Registered General Nurses*
3. Rhodes, Philip *The Value of Medicine* George Allen and Unwin, 1976 P.41
4. Rhodes, Philip op. cit. P.53
5. Rhodes, Philip op. cit. P.91
6. Council for the Education and Training of Health Visitors *An Investigation into the Principles of Health Visiting* 1977 P. 30
7. Campbell, Alastair V. *Medicine, Health, and Justice The Problem of Priorities* Churchill Livingstone P. 46
8. Campbell, Alistair V. op. cit. P. 49
9. Henderson, Virginia op. cit. P. 17

Chapter 4

A Sociologist's View of Health Visiting

Susan Willis

It is an understandable, though nor necessarily creditable aspiration for a profession to seek to establish and maintain intellectual credibility by the development of a body of literature, the exclusive nature of which is guaranteed and exemplified by its special language. Professionals have on occasions laid themselves open to the charge that they use jargon with intent to obfuscate rather than to clarify. The extensive two-way traffic between social scientists and the people they study has enabled sociologists to make frequent and often unacknowledged use of ideas and information current in society, with a familar result. The individuals or groups under such scrutiny are offered their own commonplaces as the latest discoveries of science.

A superficial examination of the principles of health visiting identifies two possible lines of approach - inquiry or indictment, but before these possibilities are explored, it is necessary to attempt some definition of the subject areas. Health visiting if it is to be a meaningful activity presumably presupposes a definition of health. The difficulties encountered when trying to encapsulate the concept of health in a succinct phrase are well known, but for the purpose of this paper, good health is taken to mean the ability to adapt to a changing environment. An absolutist definition based on physical parameters is inappropriate since it ignores the subjective elements of a state of well-being.

I have chosen to identify the primary role of the health visitor as that of enabling individuals to make their own choices about health matters. Thus, they are charged with the responsibility of facilitating self-health control. This perspective provides a comfortable and possibly comforting view of a professional activity, but is a useful position from which to begin.

The sociological contribution to the principles upon which health visiting is based may be approached by reference to, and examination of, the five part definition of the work, published by the Council for the Education and

Training of Health Visitors. The prevention of mental, physical and emotional ill health and its consequences; early detection of ill health and the surveillance of high risk groups; recognition and identification of need and mobilisation of appropriate resources where necessary; health teaching; provision of care which will include support during periods of stress and advice and guidance in illness, as well as in the care and management of young children.

Examination of the first criterion suggests that it invests health visiting with a prescriptive capacity which it clearly does not possess. It follows that since there is no precise definition of health, notions of normality and abnormality are similarly problematic. The recognition of health is an obvious prerequisite of the ability to spot deviations from it. The interpretation of perceived deviations from the normal by the individual may not be congruent with those of the health visitor and people's expectations of health may be shaped by these encounters. The demand for health may be equated directly with the demand for health care.

The early detection of ill health and the surveillance of high risk groups, coupled with the recognition and identification of need and mobilisation of appropriate resources where necessary, calls into question the nature and status of health needs.

Bradshaw, in his "Taxonomy of Social Need" (1972) identifies **normative** needs as those which are defined by the expert or professional, administrator or social scientist in any given situation. A felt need is equated with a perceived lack, or want. The **expressed** need is a felt need turned into action. The dimensions of **comparative** need are determined by studying the characteristics of a population in receipt of a service. If there are people with similar characteristics who are not receiving the service, they are in need. Ivan Illich identifies externally attributed need as a disabling effect of professions but suggests that this could not occur unless people were already experiencing as a deficiency, a lack of that which the expert imputes to them as a need. To become ignorant or unconvinced of one's own health needs has become an unforgivable social act. The worthy citizen imputes needs to himself with such conviction that desires for alternatives become repressed and the renunciation of need becomes impossible. The translation of a need into a deficiency may be identified by the sociologist as part of the strategy underpinning the power structure of the health visitor/ client relationship. Health visitors may wish to be regarded as agents of social change if the enabling perspective is adopted. An alternative view, one which is much less comfortable for the practitioner, shows the health visitor as an agent of social control. Both of these positions represent the extremes of a continuum. It is hoped that the reality lies somewhere towards the centre.

The social concomitants of illness begin with diagnosis, that is, labelling with a disease name. This is followed by a declaration of membership of a defined group, the sick, followed by the assumption of the sick role, on the part of the patient. Multiple patient status has become a sign of desirable rather than deviant behaviour, according to this perspective. To be an active client of several health care professionals confers a clearly defined place within the realm of service consumers for whom society operates. Such professional dominance facilitates economic organisation to cater for the unhealthy and their advisers/carers. The role of the health visitor as a referral agent may be seen to be rooted in the medicalisation of health and the development of specialisation. The client becomes understood and processed as a set of manageable parts.

Need defining research abounds. The available tool (remedy) defines the problem where the professional definition of need is dominant. Recent "tool using" (Illich) phenomena with which the health visitor is involved include child abuse, developmental delay and maternal deprivation.

A consideration of the concept of consumer sovereignty is important in any assessment of the principles underlying health visiting. Consumer sovereignty dictates that the individual being affected by any project planned for him is considered to be the best judge of its value. Any type of cost-benefit analysis of the worth of health teaching should aim to identify and quantify a value to the recipient. A Benthamite utilitarian dimension is shown as an important by-product of health teaching when individuals are encouraged (coerced) to take care of their own health not merely for its own sake, but to prevent them from endangering the health of others.

Any attempt to undertake effective surveillance of high risk groups presupposes the ability and the right to identify and define the areas of concern. Theories of the structure of societies based on social conflict and change identify in health teaching an element of coercion which may be present simply at the level of imposing various constraints on the degree of ignorance of a population about the risk levels they face. A liberal approach argues that by leaving individuals free to determine the values to be placed on benefits that might accrue from health enhancing behaviour we are allowing them freedom to express their preferences in decision making. This decision making process will include both an objective and a subjective assessment of risk (not necessarily recognised as such by the individuals) and of the possible cost to health of taking a chance. The sociologist would enquire whether it is correct to assume that individuals will be prepared to accept the state's (or its agents) judgements concerning the estimation of health risks as being in the best interests of the client and therefore containable within the bounds of consumer sovereignty.

For example, if a woman is told that excessive cigarette smoking in pregnancy will harm her baby (and a list of effects damaging to the fetus is explained in easy assimilable terms) in deciding whether or not to continue smoking she will almost certainly accept the judgement of the obstetrician. Indeed, although she may try to minimise the risk in her own mind she will, nevertheless, appreciate being told by an expert just what the statistically objective level of risk is. This is an area in which naked coercion fades into acceptable paternalism. If however, this judgement is wrong and paternalism is despised, the assessment is seen as a disreputable attempt to invest the argument with undeserved respectability.

The facilitation of health enhancing activities is the goal of the health visitor in health teaching. Health education may be summarised as that which ought to be done in order to bring about an improvement in health status. It is clear that individuals may exercise sanctions and initiate change to greater effect if more knowledge is held. We classify people according to the social positions which they occupy and make judgements about their actions in the light of the expectations we have about the way people occupying those positions ought to behave. Thus there are those who advocate the use of the social insurance and/or tax structure to penalise persons with poor health behaviour. Those who postulate the supremacy of naive free will, a liassez-faire attitude to health ignore, or are unaware of the complexity of human behaviour and the socio-cultural and environmental constraints on it. Thus it may be argued from this perspective that political power rests not in a monopoly of the legitimate means of violence, but in the control of information.

Enablers will use health teaching to maximise potential and to facilitate freedom of choice in the client by presenting a range of alternatives from which a reasoned choice may be made. The social controller will see the major benefit of health education as that of minimising the inconvenience and expense to the state which arises from self inflicted injury. The sociologist identifies some health education offered by the agents of the state as an ideological diversion intended to pacify the environmental health lobby, without killing the goose that lays the golden egg. Health teaching on the adverse effects of cigarette smoking and excessive alcohol consumption are included here.

The question of the credibility of the communicator assumes greater importance in the teaching of health matters especially when the aim is not merely to inform, but to influence and to change behaviour. The recipient of health teaching, if the message is to have the effect intended by the practitioner, needs to be convinced of the validity of certain claimed cause and effect relationships. Attitudes derived from norms and values may either coalesce or clash and the appropriate behavioural intention will only materialise if certain enabling factors are present. Thus, if the environment is unfavourable or hostile the desired health action will not emerge. Further, if the relevant skills or knowledge are not made available, compliance may be impossible despite high motivation. Thus both the medium and the message must be acceptable for effective health teaching.

The function of the health visitor in the provision of care to include support during periods of stress and advice on the management of children cloaks potent political symbolism with an aura of loving protection. In modern industrial society where the service industries predominate, the economic reality identifies as essential, adequate financial support for health care workers and the services they offer. The important principle of health attainment and maintenance by individuals and families themselves in preventing disease and accidents without the intervention of the health visitor or paramedical professional should not however be disregarded.

A sociology contribution to principles in practice attempts to discover some of the methods by which consumers may question health care. Apathy is not regarded as a valid indicator of satisfaction. The criteria to be met in establishing and maintaining a worthwhile system of health care and teaching should be based on acceptability, accessibility, availability, continuity, low cost (to the recipient) and high quality. The level of acceptability will vary directly with the level of utilisation. The expectations which the consumer may have about a system of health care planning may be at variance with those of the practitioners. Reaching all segments of the population with preventive care has always been difficult. Slesinger, in his study of the utilisation of preventive medical services published in 1973, concluded that acceptance of preventive medical care varies, in statistical terms, directly with socio-economic status and a positive medical orientation and inversely with social isolation. Differences in social class influences produce differential perception and responses to illness. Similarly the class and culture-bound character of professional attitudes makes value free judgements about their clients impossible. This distinction is often identified as a causative factor in the oppressive nature of some health visitor/client relationships.

The contribution of the sociological perspective to the knowledge base of health visiting may be explored through several theoretical approaches. Max Weber's distinction between social and non-social action has been the precursor of many later sociological theories. He defined social action as action "orientated towards the past, present or expected future behaviour of others". The others may constitute an indefinite plurality. The salient features of this type of social action theory which makes an ideal vehicle for an exploration of health visiting principles, are these. The actor has goals, or aims and his actions are carried out in pursuit of these. Action often involves the selection of means directed towards the attainment of goals. An actor may have multiple goals; actions in pursuit of any one affect and are affected by those in pursuit of others. Certain assumptions are made by the actor concerning the nature of the goals and the possibility of their attainment. The actor has certain affective tendencies which affect both his perception of situations and the choice of goals. Entrenched norms and values also govern the selection of goals and their ranking in order of priority.

A social-psychological approach to the principles of health visiting involves a study of individuals in interaction and in relation to their social environment. Usually, the family provides the individual's earliest social environment and studies of patterns of socialisation and child rearing techniques to include feeding, toilet training and control strategies, make a valuable contribution. The acquisition of language and mechanisms for exploring and controlling conflict and for engendering cooperation among family members provide fascinating insights into these complex yet fluid structures. The concept of role is fundamental to any analysis in social-psychological terms because it enables an individual's behaviour to be defined in terms of a relevant, current social environment. This perspective, when applied to the priniciples of health visiting may, for example, seek to identify high levels of unmet needs in a given population and is related to the ways by which people determine their need for help with health care.

A further implication of normative need described earlier is that if it is indeed subject to definition only by a third party, one who is external to the individual in need, there must exist some indicator or observable characteristic which provides the basic information necessary for the identification and assessment of need. The identification of unmet needs represents a serious waste of professional and economic resources and exploits human uncertainty and distress if misapplied. For example, some screening procedures are morally questionable if no treatment for the identified disorder is either available or effective.

Demographic studies may be used to quantify variations in the uses made of the health visiting service and can be related to age, sex, occupation, ethnicity, fertility and socio-economic status. The term fertility is used by demographers to indicate actual reproductive performance, as distinct from fecundity which is defined as the physiological capacity to reproduce. Any study of fertility clearly illustrates a societal interest in the control of reproduction and in the nature of marriage patterns. Care should be taken when using this approach that the social categories do not become perjorative labels which may then be used to reinforce already damaging stereotypes.

A recent and evolving sociological perspective which makes a significant contribution to a study of the principles of health visiting, albeit by a somewhat esoteric and possibly inadvertent route, is ethnomethodology. The ethnomethodologist directs attention to the question of how a social order is possible. Garfunkel's work in 1976 takes as its primary concern, analysis of the routine, taken-for-granted expectations that the members of any social order accept regularly. The form and nature of these expectations constitute the central focus of ethnomethodology. Much recent work serves to amplify the research of social interactionists on the labelling process. For example, Becker postulates that deviance does not reside in social acts but must be traced to definitions which arise during interaction. The significance of this approach for health education techniques will be recognised. The ethnomethodologist has blended a concern with deviance with the study of social organisation and social relationships. For example, an organisational structure approach may be used to account for differential health and illness behaviour when the structure of the system established for the delivery of health care is examined.

Finally, a system approach provides models which may, or may not be ideal typical, which can be used to explicate causal structures and incorporate features of all the other theoretical perspectives to obtain new insights into the principles upon which the discipline of health visiting is founded. A social system is defined as comprising two or more individuals acting directly or indirectly in a bounded situation. The fundamental sociological point of reference is that the participants are orientated to a common focus or interrelated foci. Emphasis on the normative regulation of behaviour and a preoccupation with integrative phenomena have produced the criticism that the systems theorist is blind to the reality and the value of dissent and conflict in everyday life.

The early relationship of health visiting to sociology may be described as coincidental, or even fortuitous, but the current situation is neither of these. Since man is both a social and a political animal, the priniciples of health visiting must be based upon a knowledge of the prevailing social structure, its composition in terms of the nature, proportions and diversities of the various groups contained within it and the power relationships which operate in the management of competing claims for scarce resources. These features constitute some of the prime concerns of the enterprise of sociology today and Mitchell suggests that the discipline has become one of the major forms of our self-awareness in the twentieth century.

Clearly, if a profession is to survive it must develop and its knowledge base must grow. Appropriate questions must be asked, relevant problems examined and valid, workable conclusions drawn in order that credibility may be maintained. It is hoped that it has been shown that the contribution of sociology to this professional development and to the priniciples upon which health visiting is based is not peripheral, but central.

Bibliography

1. BECKER H A : *Outsiders*, 1963 Collier Macmillan
2. BENDIX R & LIPSET S M : *Class Status and Power*, 1953 Routledge and Kegan Paul
3. BENN S I & PETER R S : *Social Principles and the Democratic State*, 1959 Allen and ßunwin
4. BOTTOMORE T B : *Sociology - A Guide to Problems and Literature*, 1962 Allen and Unwin
5. BOTTOMORE T & NISBET R (EDITORS) : *A History of Sociological Analysis*, 1978 Heinemann
6. BRADSHAW : *Taxonomy of Social Need*, 1972 In McLachlan Problems and Progress in Medical Care, Oxford University Press
7. DAHRENDORF R : *Out of utopia - Towards a reorientation of Sociological Analysis*, 1958 American Journal of Sociology September 1958 P112-116
8. GARFINKEL H : Studies in Ethnomethodology, 1967 Prentice-Hall
9. GERTH H & MILLS C W : *From Max Weber - Essays in Sociology*, 1947 Kegan Paul
10. GIDDENS A : *Capitalism and Modern Social Theory - An Analysis of the Writings of Marx*, Durkehim and Max Weber, 1971 Cambridge University Press
11. ILLICH I ET AL : *Disabling Professions*, 1977 Marion Bowers
12. MERTON R K : *Social Theory and Social Structure*, 1957 The Free Press
13. PARSONS T : *The Social System*, 1952 Tavistock Publications
14. RADCLIFFE—BROWN A R : *Structure and Function in Primitive Society*, 1952 Cohen and West
15. MITCHELL G D : *A Dictionary of Sociology*, 1968 Routledge and Kegan Paul
16. CETHV : *The Function of The Health Visitor*

Chapter 5

Theory into Practice - The Health Visitor Course as a Preparation for the Reality of Practice

Alison McClymont

Introduction

In **Teaching for Reality** (McClymont 1980) it was demonstrated that although 96% of the qualified health visitors in the sample expressed the opinion that they had found the health visitor course either useful or very useful as a preparation for their role in practice, 76% of the group had found it necessary to change their perception of their role as a health visitor following qualification. In the conclusions to the study this apparent conflict in the findings was rationalised by the observation that "in spite of the necessity for role change or adjustment after qualification, the course was wide enough, and flexible enough, to have been of use as preparation for the changing and changed perceptions of role".

The sample used for the study comprised fifty health visitors who had qualified during the previous five years (1972-1977) from two health visitor courses. The findings relate to this study only but are worthy of review, and challenge by other course leaders in other areas of the United Kingdom.

During the data collecting stage of the study differing aspects of the course were criticised and subject expansion and subject changes were suggested,

    eg. "more periods needed to be spent working in specialist areas and handicaps in general".

        "greater detail regarding cultural patterns with immigrant population and their special problems".

Other members of the sample expressed contentment with the course,

    eg. "The course was relevant and has helped in my day to day health visiting. I have been surprised at how useful some of the information gained in the course has been".

        "I still feel we must be taught the ideal in College and learn from experience in our own area after that".

These two latter opinions express the sentiments of many respondents and they also coincide with the view of the CETHV's Working Group on the Principles of Health Visiting

"Principles should assist in teaching, evaluating and in providing an ideal module. Although we are fully aware of the difference in many instances between what is taught and what is or can be practised, we believe that the ideal provides a comparison for the ordering of reality, so as to achieve the best possible outcome". (CETHV 1977)

Recognition that no course can ever be perfect for all participants is one way out of this situation but it cannot be adopted as the ultimate excuse for ever. Although it may be comforting for course organisers to find that 96% of those attending found the course useful or very useful, it should be equally disturbing to them to find that 76% of those attending required adaptation to practice after qualification.

These findings lead to questions which deserve exploration and explanation. What is taught? What is practised? Where and how do the two meet? Could there be improvement?

What is taught?

What are the subjects covered in the health visitor course and how were these decided upon?

The Council for the Training of Health Visitors* set the syllabus with its five sections,

the development of the individual,
the individual in the group,
the development of social policy,
the social aspects of health and disease,
the principles and practice of health visiting,

for implementation in the new style health visitor courses commencing in 1965.

The need for a change in syllabus and a change in outlook regarding health visiting came from the Report of the Working Party on the field of work, training and recruitment of health visitors under the chairmanship of Sir Wilson Jameson. The Report, published in 1956 under the title "An Inquiry into Health Visiting" stated

"Witnesses' criticsms of the existing courses are to the effect that they are too short, too crammed, too theoretical and too little concerned with

* Established in 1965 as the Council for the Training of Health Visitors, the Council's title was changed in 1972 to the Council for the Education and Training of Health Visitors

modern views on psychological aspects and family relationships. There is said to be a tendency to repeat matter covered in previous training. The range of subjects on which students may be examined is so wide that the training centres are said to be over much concerned with preparing students for an academic examination rather than with giving them a sound practical professional education. The nature and manner of providing practical experience has been singled out for criticism by some." (Para. 352)

"Generally, we think that the objects of training should be two: firstly, to provide the health visitor with the essential additional technical knowledge that she immediately needs for her own work and, secondly, to give her a clear picture of family welfare services and her part in them. No attempt should be made to give the student the full range of knowledge that an experienced health visitor has. It is enough that she should know principles well and where to look for further help as an when the need arises. ..." (Para. 353)

The Council stated that their objectives for training were twofold:-
"First the assessment of the health potential of the individual and family group and provision of appropriate health education; and, second, assessing the health needs of the handicapped of all age groups, the implication of their care on the family and their continued maintenance and support in the community". (CTHV 1965),
and the syllabus was designed with the objectives and working environment in mind to:-
"a) sharpen the students capacity to perceive early deviations from the normal;
b) give her knowledge of various statutory and voluntary agencies which may assist in any particular family situation;
c) provide practice in the working out of a programme of help for the individual where this is required;
d) prepare her to select the method of health education likely to be the most successful in any particular instance." (CTHV 1965)

The syllabus which emerged from these thoughts and deliberations has formed the basis of health visitor courses since 1965. Within the broad syllabus flexibility has been found by the staffs of the many institutions holding health visitor courses and although there is a commonality within all courses, in that there must be syllabus coverage under CETHV regulations for course approval, each course is different. CETHV does not lay down specific subject criteria within the syllabus, or within the sections of the syllabus, therefore every course has developed according to the needs of the community the course serves, and according to the expertise and experience of the staff serving the course.

What is practised?

What is the role of the health visitor? This question always draws a response of puzzlement from both within and outwith the profession that the questioner does not know the answer, yet the odds are that on scrutiny each respondent's answer would be found to differ from every other respondent's answer. Why is this so? It has been suggested that it is because health visitors are themselves uncertain of what they do (Hunt 1972) or that they have allowed others to dictate what they do (Rehin 1972), or that the role is so wide that no one person could perform it (Hicks 1976).

In 1969 the Report of the Working Party on Management Structure in the Local Authority Nursing Service (Mayston Report) gave a full job description for the health visitor. Hicks (1976) later described this as "a cruel burden of responsibility to impose on anyone .... by any method of counting (it) is a formidable list requiring a wide-ranging knowledge and rare gifts of presentation and persuasion".

In 1974 the Chief Nursing Officer to the Department of Health and Social Security sent a letter to the newly appointed Regional, Area and District Nursing Officers "describing the present scope and possible future direction" of the health visiting (and home nursing) services. The Mayston Report formed the basis of these descriptions but their format is more readable.

The health visiting service is described thus.:-
".... health visitors have assisted local health authorities to discharge their responsibilities under the NHS Act 1946 and the Health Services and Public Health Act 1968 for:
1. care of expectant and nursing mothers and young children;
2. prevention of illness and promotion of health;
3. care and after care of persons suffering or who have suffered from illness;
4. medical and dental inspection and treatment of school children;
5. health education;
6. family planning.
Their functions in these fields, which will not be affected by NHS reorganisation, have broadly been as follows:
1. **Care of expectant and nursing mothers and young children** - The **health visitor** is often involved at ante-natal clinics, young wives'

clubs, mothers' clubs etc. in group teaching on parenthood, spacing
of births and prevention of unwanted pregnancies. In co-operation
with the midwife, the health visitor arranges to see each mother and
her baby at home to ensure that any necessary continuing help and
care is provided when the midwife's responsibilities cease. The health
visitor is concerned to detect at an early stage signs of physical or
mental abnormality in the young child. She participates with the
general practitioner of health authority doctor in running child health
clinics. It is part of her function to know and visit all young children,
especially those known to be at risk. She maintains health records of
these children and ensures that relevant health information is passed
on to the school authorities at the appropriate time. Her records can
also be made available to other members of the primary health care
team - general practitioner, home nurse etc.

2. **Prevention of illness** - The **health visitor** has a special responsibility
   for the prevention of illness in all members of a family. Because she
   visits families before and after the birth of a baby she is ideally
   placed to recognise and identify potential hazards to health in the
   home, and to assess the danger of stress within the family or in social
   relationships. The health visitor comes into contact with many people
   through her work in health education - in schools, ante-natal clinics,
   old peoples' clubs, etc. She is often involved also in the follow-up of
   of persons known or believed to be suffering from sexually transmitted diseases, in screening programmes, and in prophylaxis.
   Health visitors attached to general practice, at health centres or
   elsewhere, are exceptionally well placed to provide or, by referral, to
   secure health advice or other support to potentially vulnerable
   groups, such as the elderly, mentally ill or physically or mentally
   handicapped, and people who are newly bereaved or living alone.

3. **Care of persons suffering from illness.** The visiting of patients
   suffering from tuberculosis is a health visiting function carried out in
   some areas by specialist **tuberculosis visitors** employed for this
   purpose.

4. **After-care of patients who have been ill.** The **health visitor** may be
   called upon to take part, in conjunction with other professional
   colleagues, in assessing the needs of patients who are about to be
   admitted to or discharged from hospital. The **health visitor** provides
   or arranges any necessary advice and support for the patient and/or
   his family.

5. **Medical and dental inspection and treatment of school children.** The **health visitor** in her capacity as school nurse has responsibilities for the care of school children including handicapped pupils. She participates as necessary in school medical inspections, screening tests for sight and hearing, immunisation clinics and health education classes. She keeps appropriate records and works as necessary with the children's teachers, educational authorities, families and general practitioners. She has special responsibilities for the handicapped child.

6. **Family planning services** - The **health visitor's** role in family planning is to ensure that all mothers are made aware of the available services to help them in the spacing of families and avoiding unwanted pregnancies. Advice and help may be given by health visitors at ante-natal teaching sessions, during visits to mothers in hospital in the lying-in period or when visiting mothers in their own homes. Occasions arise when the health visitor is able to assist young persons in need of family planning advice. The health visitor is able to refer those people requiring advice on contraception to the appropriate clinic or general practitioner.

Future Scope of the Services

In recent years considerable developments have taken place in the provision of nursing services outside hospital notably in respect of home nursing and health visiting services and schemes of attachment with general practice. One effect of these developments has been to extend the scope and volume of the work of home nurses and health visitors as part of primary health care. It is in connection with work associated with the elderly, the physically and mentally handicapped, the mentally ill and other vulnerable groups, and in meeting the additional work involved in treating more patients outside hospital and the early discharge of hospital patients, that the functions of the nursing services in primary health care have been changing and expanding. Future areas of concern are likely to include:

1. **The Prevention of illness**
   a. **Health education** of the public in such matters as sexual relationships, contraception, smoking, sexually transmitted diseases, alcoholism, drug addiction and obesity is likely to develop in importance.
   b. **Screening.** Health visitors will play an increasing part in health screening of children (early identification of handicap), and in cervical and bladder cytology and in early tracing of contacts with venereal and other sexually transmitted diseases.

    c. **Case Finding.** Identifying and visiting deprived families and other families 'at risk' by health visitors and other members of the primary health care team is likely to increase in parallel with special continuing efforts to ensure that full use is made of the child health services.

2. **Long term care for special health care groups.** Many people who are ill, infirm through age or other causes, permanently handicapped or dying would prefer to be cared for at home rather than in a hospital or residential institution. Extra work will fall upon the home nursing, health visiting and personal social services if such wishes are to be met.

3. **Selective care and treatment.** The current trend is away from routine medical and dental inspection and treatment of school children towards a 'selective' approach and follow-up of individual pupils in need of care.

4. **Family planning services.** The spread of domiciliary family planning services will involve the health visitor in further work in seeking out and educating in their own homes those women most at risk of an unwanted pregnancy but who do not avail themselves of the services provided at clinics and other centres. Some health visitors and home nurses will need specialised training to enable them to undertake clinical duties alongside a doctor either at the clinic or general practitioner surgery.''

This outline or description by the CNO/DHSS demonstrates the enormity of the task set for the health visitor. The scope for promotion of health and prevention of ill health throughout the population is almost limitless. As health visitors have moved into primary health care teams, based in health centres the population they are expected to serve has become the total population and the role they are expected to play is that of all things to all men, women and children included, in the field of health education. The areas of work outlined in the section above 'future scope of the services' have made increasing inroads into the more traditional role in the previous section.

Where and how do theory and practice meet?

The study which formed the basis of **Teaching for Reality** set out specifically to review this question. The purpose of this study was to observe whether the health visitor course put forward a realistic usable theory for the role of the health visitor, or whether the theory of the course proved in practice to be an espoused theory, which the students upon qualification would find incompatible with the practical theory-in-use. (For detail of theory, espoused theory and theory-in-use see Argyris and Schon 1974).

The findings of the study demonstrate that overall the qualified health visitors responded very positively in their opinion of the usefulness of the health visitor course as a preparation for the role of health visitor.

Table 1 Overall opinion of the usefulness of the health visitor course as a preparation for the role of health visitor

Qualified Health Visitors	Very Useful	Useful	Undecided	Not very useful	Useless
50	11	37	1	1	—

It cannot escape notice that the majority had found the course useful rather than very useful, indicating that improvement of the course and its application to practice would be possible.

To review which area of the course the respondents found most useful/least useful it is necessary to break down the syllabus into subject areas. This analysis is most interesting as it indicates the spread of content/discontent or satisfaction/dissatisfaction with the differing aspects of the course.

The most useful subjects of the course in the health visitors' opinion were those which once they had qualified they could use right away - the 'here and now' subjects. The areas of study which required application to practice were found least useful, though it must be most strongly emphasised no subject area in the syllabus was viewed as totally unnecessary as even the lowest scored subject area was viewed as useful by 52% of the health visitors.

Could there be improvement?

The short answer to "could there be improvement"? must be yes. There are bases for improvement in the teaching, in the practice and in the relationship between the theory and practice of health visiting.

Table 2 Comparison of the opinion of usefulness of the differing aspects of the course.

	VU	U	Und	NvU	Us
Section I. Development of the Individual					
(i) Psychology	23	17	4	5	1
(ii) Physiological development	35	13	2	-	-
(iii) Nutrition	28	17	2	3	-
(iv) Genetics	12	31	3	2	2
(v) Development of the special senses	28	16	5	-	1
Section II. The individual in the Group					
(i) Sociology lectures	16	23	3	4	4
(ii) Seminars in Sociology	6	20	8	11	5
(iii) Sociology discussion groups	10	20	6	9	5
Section III. Development of Social Policy					
(i) Development of health & social services	5	34	3	8	-
(ii) Current health & Social Services	26	22	-	2	-
(iii) Services for handicapped/deprived	34	9	5	2	-
(iv) The school health services	17	23	4	6	-
(v) Occupational health	2	26	12	10	-
Section IV. Social Aspects health/disease					
(i) Health Statistics	8	23	10	6	3
(ii) Epidemiology and Infectious disease	15	27	3	4	1
(iii) Aspects of Community Medicine	16	28	5	-	1
(iv) Handicap ... physical	32	15	1	2	-
mental illness	27	16	2	5	-
mental handicap	33	12	2	3	-
(v) Immigrant Health	13	21	9	6	1
(vi) Geriatrics and Rehabilitation	16	25	5	3	1
Section V. Principles & Practice of H. Visiting					
(i) Health visiting theory/role/function	27	20	2	1	-
(ii) HV practice ... problems/studies	30	12	3	5	-
(iii) Health Education	22	21	3	4	-
(iv) Nursing/Health Visiting Law	9	29	5	6	1
(v) Observation Visits	18	18	5	9	-
(vi) Fieldwork placement	30	14	1	4	1
(vii) Alternative practice	20	18	5	6	1
(viii) Supervised practice	39	8	1	1	1

This analysis demonstrates that although the students had found the course useful as a whole, there were some subject areas which they had found more useful than others, and conversely some they had found less usefull then others. A comparison of the ranked order of usefulness of the subject areas provides food for thought.

Table 3 Rank order of opinion of subject components of the syllabus by student sample.
(Twenty-four components covered by lecture programme)

Ranked in order- most useful to least useful	Useful Per Cent	Not Useful Per Cent
1. Current health and social services	96	4
2. Physiological development	96	4
3. Physical handicap	94	6
4. Health visiting theory and role	94	6
5. Mental handicap	90	10
6. Nutrition	90	10
7. Community medicine	88	12
8. Development of Special Senses	88	12
9. Health education	86	14
10. Mental illness	86	14
11. Services for Handicaps	86	14
12. Genetics	86	14
13. Epidemiology	84	16
14. Geriatrics	82	18
15. School health	80	20
16. Psychology	80	20
17. Development of Social Policy	78	22
18. Sociology lectures	78	22
19. Nursing and Health visiting law	76	24
20. Immigrant health	68	32
21. Health statistics	62	38
22. Sociology discussion groups	60	40
23. Occupational health	56	44
24. Sociology seminars	52	48

Table 4 Rank order of opinion of subject components of the syllabus by student sample. Five components covered by theory to practice

Ranked in order most useful to least useful	Useful Per Cent	Not Useful Per Cent
1. Supervised practice	94	6
2. Fieldwork teaching	88	12
3. Health Visiting Practice - Studies	84	16
4. Alternative practice	76	24
5. Observation visits	72	28

The qualified health visitors in the study which led to **Teaching for Reality** identified, through their responses, the subject area which they found least useful to them in their application of theory to practice. These were the subjects which lacked the 'here and now' factor of the most useful subjects. The least useful were the subjects which could not be related directly to the everyday experiences of the health visitor.

Knowles (1977) puts forward the view that adults generally are not interested in storing information, they are interested in the 'here and now' in putting into practice, at the latest 'tomorrow' what they are learning 'today'. They are interested in learning what will help them improve the quality of their lives, and their work; what will aid promotion. When this is related to a health visitor course it could be seen in an almost direct relationship to the students on the course. There is no research finding which relates directly to student health visitor intake ambitions, but it could be postulated that many students enter the course in order to improve the quality of their lives and to aid their promotion prospects. They are interested in the here and now, in the reality of their own world. Teaching which does not fit into this scheme will not necessarily be rejected, but will not be as readily utilised as teaching which does.

Dingwell (1977) in his study of health visitor students found that any subject which has an analytical approach rather than a "commonsensical" approach was "quite unintelligible to students who preferred teaching which extended the ideas they brought with them".

In studies on the subject of adult learning this is a common theme. Adults are interested in the here and now. The amount of experience a person has may be utilized as a base to build upon, may be a rich source of knowledge, understanding, know-how, and from the foundation stone of further learning and discovery. Or, it may form a stable or static base to be withheld at all costs! "Older people (over 35) tend to have great difficulty in accepting new ideas, methods, concepts and principles, It is as if they are handicapped by what they already know and believe. And so they appear rigid and unyielding." (Davies 1971). Cooper (1977) voices this same point of view, i.e. that adults are creatures of habit; that they are set in their ways and thinking; that many experienced nurses repeat procedures taught in their training schools throughout their professional lives regardless of new or innovative thoughts on the matter. If this is the case, within any health visitor course there must be a built in period of unfreezing or opening up. A time for experienced nurses to become aware that the health visitor course does require re-learning as no individual can overcome a problem of rigidity or stasis if they are unaware they have it.

In the practice of health visiting there are wide variations of function performed and of role expectancy. In the **Teaching for Reality** study it was demonstrated that health visitors employed by differing health authorities emphasised different aspects of their role, regardless of the teaching of the health visitor course. It was also postulated that because of the shortage of health visiting manpower the various authorities had chosen different priorities of the role for the service in their Areas. With a job description as broad and wide as that outlined in the Mayston Report (1969) and with health visitors serving a population of 1 : 4,500 - 7,500 (in the study areas) rather than the 1 : 3-4,600 recommended by the government departments in 1972 the full role cannot always be achieved and priorities must be set. In 1973 Clark studied health visiting in Berkshire and set out to try to clarify the content of the home visit of the health visitor. Within her conclusions she stated 'it may be possible for a health visitor in Aberdeen, responsible for a population of 2,500 to adopt the role of an all purpose family visitor; for a health visitor in Ealing, responsible for a population of 15,700 it is clearly impossible to do so''.

The situation in both Aberdeen and Ealing is in all likelihood different now, but the message remains the same. Health visitors can only do so much. If the job description is wide, and the number of health visitors small the service given will not meet the presumptions of those who accept complete coverage of the role.

Health visiting is a generalist, not a specialist service. Each course must prepare health visitors for work in general, for work in any part of the United Kingdom, not for work in any specific area or venue. Course leaders should always take cognizance of relevant research findings, both within the field of health visiting as well as within adult and general education. Courses should be innovative and newly qualified staff should be regarded as a constant updating element within the health care team and within the health visiting service yet this will only be achieved if the health visitor courses remain in contact with practice.

Course leaders and service managers should continue to work together to achieve a situation in which theory and practice develop together to the benefit of the service and profession.

BIBLIOGRAPHY

ARGYRIS, C., SCHON, D.A. (1974)
Theory in Practice: Increasing professional effectiveness.
Jossey-Bass, San Francisco.

CLARK, June (1973)
  A Family Visitor
  RCN London
COOPER, S.S. and HORNBACK, M.S. (1973)
  Continuing Nursing Education
  McGraw Hill Book Company, New York
CTHV (1965) *Background to the syllabus of training*
CETHV (1977) *An Investigation into the Principles of Health Visiting*
DAVIES, I.K. (1971)
  The management of learning
  McGraw Hill Book Company, New York
DHSS (1969) *Report of the Working Party on Management Structure in Local Authority
      Nursing Services*
      Chairman, E. L. Mayston
      DHSS London
DHSS (1972) *Local Health Authority Circular 13/72*
DHSS (1974) *Home Nursing and Health Visiting Services - CNO Letter - E/C232/4*
SHHD (1972) *Local Health Authority Circular 10/72*
DINGWALL, Robert (1977)
  The Social Organisation of Health Visitor Training
  Croom Helm, London.
HICKS, Donald (1976)
  Primary Health Care
  HMSO London
HUNT, Maura (1972)
  The dilemma of identity in health visiting.
  Nursing Times, Vol. 68, Occasional Papers 3 Feb. pp 17-20
                                        10 Feb. pp 23-24
KNOWLES, M. S. (1977)
  Gearing adult education to the seventies
  In Popiel, E.S. (Ed) (1977) Nursing and the process of Continuing Education
  C.V. Mosby Company, Saint Louis
McCLYMONT, A. (1980)
  Teaching for Reality
  CETHV London
MINISTRY OF HEALTH (1956)
  An inquiry into health visiting
  Chairman, W. Jameson
  H.M.S.O. London
REHIN, G.F. (1972)
  The 'Point and Purpose' of the health visitor.
  Nursing Times, Vol. 68, pp 304-307

Chapter 6

A Case Study in Methodology
Job satisfaction in Health Visiting - How can it be measured?

Pat Ellis

The aim of this chapter is to present some questionnaire techniques which may be used in looking at various aspects of work. Increasingly, members of the health visiting profession are faced with the need or desire to examine areas of their work or profession in a systematic manner. These investigations may come about as the result of demands of an academic course with its 'project' or from pressures at work. Some studies may be classified as full blown research ventures with one or more persons involved over a considerable length of time. Whatever the scope and size of the study, one of the major decisions that always has to be considered and often causes problems is that of choosing appropriate methods of data collection. Examples in this chapter are taken from a study of job satisfaction amongst health visitors (Ellis, 1980).

1. The Aims of the Health Visitor Research

During the 1960s growing fears were being expressed in the health visiting profession that there was a high level of dissatisfaction in the profession and that this was leading to an unacceptably high drop-out rate from the occupation. Such fears had first been mentioned in the Jameson Report (1956). Although little research was done in this area, the unease being expressed was centred around the ill-defined nature of the role of the health visitor and the acceptance of the health visitor by the other caring occupations working within the community. At the same time the 1960s had seen the inauguration of what is now the Council for the Education and Training of Health Visitors followed by the introduction in 1965 of a new national syllabus for training. This then was the background to the study 'Job Satisfaction amongst Health Visitors' carried out in the 1970s.

The aim of the research was to build a picture of how health visitors saw their work and to explore the nature of job satisfaction within health visiting. In view of the concern over level of drop-out from the profession, it was felt that it was most sensible to investigate new entrants. It was decided to follow a sample through from the time they entered their training course to the end of their first year of qualified work experience. 405 new entrants answered the first questionnaire and of these 250 remained with the research to its completion.

2. Measurement of job satisfaction : What Methods?

A search of the literature on job satisfaction, of which there is a useful summary in Locke (1976), revealed that conceptually there were two ways of considerng the topic. The first approach examined job satisfaction (JS) as an entity in itself which could be seen as an overall reaction to the job and the second approach used job facet satisfaction (JFS) which was the reactions to various facets or aspects of the work. How did this relate to looking at health visiting? It was decided that it would be valid and useful to use both approaches and so try to obtain reactions to both health visiting in general and to various parts of the work such as health education.

A serious weakness in studies conducted in this area of job satisfaction when it came to looking at health visiting was that the studies were in the main carried out:

    a. looking at men
    b. taking work in the private sector of the economy
    c. American based.

A further complication was that very few studies worked with professionally trained people who accordingly enjoyed a degree of autonomy in their occupations which is not usually present to the same extent for those who are not professionally qualified. These constraints meant that unfortunately there were not tailor-made questions that could be taken directly from previous researches and used in the study of health visiting. It was therefore a case of looking at a variety of techniques used in questionnaire design and considering those that could most usefully be incorporated into the health visiting research.

In this chapter three types of questioning techniques will be described and illustrated. These were not the only techniques used. However they are quoted because they proved especially useful in this study with each producing very different types of results and so may be of interest to the reader.

3. Basic Decisions : Methods of Data Collection

Questionnaires are frequently seen as the most useful way to collect data that will form the basis of a study. This is because they allow the researcher:

- easy contact with a large sample of potential subjects
- the possibility of a short span of time involved in collection
- a wide geographical spread of the sample
- standardisation of questions between respondents
- standardisation of questions across time

Because of these benefits, it was decided in the health visiting research to use questionnaires as the main means of data collection. Each subject ie. new entrants to health visiting was to be asked to answer three questionnaires, at the start and end of training and after one year of work. This meant that health visitors could be compared with each other for similarities and differences as well as over time for constancies and changes in response.

Two decisions then had to be made, the first on what questions should go into the questionnaires and the second on the size and composition of the sample. This latter decision is examined in the last section of the chapter.

Various question techniques were used. Three in particular are looked at because they illustrate a range of ways of collecting data and some of the options open for presentation of results. The techniques are;

    A.   open-ended questions
    B.   Likert scale statements
    C.   semantic differential scales.

A. Open-ended questions

Open-ended questions are those where the nature of the response and its length are determined by the person answering rather than by the person designing the questionnaire. Obviously, the subject area to be commented upon is outlined in the question and the length of the reply tends to be indicated by the space left on the page.

It may be the most satisfying type of question as it allows the greatest freedom of response. However, because of this it may need greater thought on the part of the respondent and consequently take longer than ticking one of several alternatives. For the researcher, the responses often yield a wealth of information but there is the danger that a proportion of it will not be of relevance to the study. Questions therefore must be well-worded and non-ambiguous to avoid as far as possible irrelevancies that arise from misunderstandings. It is sensible to test out or pilot questionnaires on a practice group to iron out such problems before embarking on the main sample. A much bigger difficulty attached to such questions is the sheer amount and spread of information generated which then needs to be analysed.

As O'Muircheartaigh (1977) points out, methods of analysis provide a means of transforming the raw survey data into a meaningful set of results. Responses to open-ended questions are a form of qualitative data in that they are words and sentences representing various ideas and types of information. Difficulties arise when trying to undertake mathematical operations such as addition, ranking and subsequent statistical manipulations on data in this form.

Content analysis is a process by which qualitative data is transformed into quantitative. It is basically a classification procedure which uses the responses to suggest the suitable classifications to adopt within the context of the research. There are two stages in this process - the first is the construction of classification categories and the second is the assignment of the responses to these categories.

All health visitors in this study had progressed to their present position through nursing.* In looking at how they saw health visiting, it was necessary to get an indication of how this transition had been made in terms of motivation and interest. In order not to constrain the responses of the sample, open-ended questions were deemed to be the most appropriate method to use. Three questions were therefore asked:

1.   What were your reasons for entering nursing?
2.   What were your reasons for leaving hospital work?
3.   What were your reasons for applying for a health visiting course?

Each of these questions produced a large number of responses. These were then broken down into separate ideas (often several per response). These ideas were examined together to see if any categories were present. Table 1 shows the categories that emerged from the responses to the first question and how these categories in turn further grouped together. Each category was assigned a code number. Research staff then went back and read each questionnaire response and allocated the relevant code numbers to indicate the content of the response. This coded data was then entered into the computer and a simple count made of the number of responses falling into each of the major categories.

Since 1965 all health visitor students are required to be SRNs.

Table 1

QUESTION 1 CODING SCHEME "What were your reasons for entering nursing".

PEOPLE—Caring, helping and meeting them

Code	Subsection heading
11	a) To nurse and care for people
12	b) To help people
13	c) Interest in people/meeting/working with people
14	d) Worthwhile job/service to others

JOB—Background, positive and negative aspirations

Code	Subsection heading	
21	a) School/YEO influence	
22	b) Medical background or interest in family	Background
23	c) Childhood ambition	
24	d) Interest in medicine/first-aid/biology	
31	e) Good career/occupation/training	+ ve job aspiration
32	f) Interesting/satisfying work	
41	g) No other job considered	
42	h) Nothing else wished to do	-ve job aspirations
43	i) Lack of alternative	
44	j) Dislike of 9-5/sedentary/office jobs	

MISCELLANEOUS

Code	Section heading
90	Miscellaneous

Table 2

*REASONS FOR ENTERING NURSING ***

Content analysis category	Full Q1 sample
Caring for, helping and meeting people	267
Family background/childhood ambition/school interest	156
Positive interest in the work	131
Nothing else considered/dislike of alternatives	73
Sample size	405

Questionnaire 1 part 1 question 1

Table 3

*REASONS FOR LEAVING HOSPITAL WORK ***

Content analysis category	Full Q1 sample
Domestic commitments	178
Internal hospital conditions	104
General dissatisfaction with hospital nursing	90
Personal reasons	13
Desire for personal/career futherance	122
Interest in social/preventive aspects of nursing	173
Sample size	405

Questionnaire 1 part 1 question 2

Table 4

REASONS FOR ENTERING HEALTH VISITING *

Content analysis category	Full Q1 sample
Domestic circumstances	114
Need or wish to move from hospital or district	31
Desire to further career or education	262
Interest in people/health education/preventive medicine	255
Sample size	405

* Questionnaire 1 part 1 question 3

Tables 2, 3 and 4 show the overall results of the content analysis of questions 1, 2 and 3. The total number of people involved in answering was 405. However, many of the sample included more than one category in their response and this is why, for example, there are 627 responses in total from the 405 in the sample to question 1.

The results in table 2 with the emphasis on caring for, helping and meeting people (66% of the sample) fit in very well with the findings of MacGuire (1966), Singh (1970) and Anderson (1973). Gradually with progression through a career, other factors appear to become important. Domestic commitments assume a prominent position in the responses and also more clearly specified approaches to work than the initial general 'humanitarianism'. Given the particular shifts in emphasis, the responses to questions 2 and 3 were further analysed to discover whether these changes were associated with the marital status of the sample. As tables 5 and 6 demonstrate, this appeared to be the case backed up by statistically significant results and confirmed what many would intuitively anticipate.

Another area of concern in the research was the way in which the health visitors viewed the make-up of their work in relation to both the contribution it makes to the community and the satisfaction it gives them. Two questions were asked in several of the questionnaires to enable a comparison to be made over time. These were:

1. Which 2 aspects of the work of the health visitor do you think make the greatest contribution to the welfare of the community?

2.   Which 2 or 3 aspects of the work of the health visitor do you expect to give you the greatest amount of satisfaction?

Table 5

REASONS FOR LEAVING HOSPITAL WORK ANALYSED BY MARITAL STATUS *

Content analysis category	MARITAL STATUS		Total
	Single	Married	
Domestic commitments	43	133	176
Internal hospital conditions	61	43	104
General dissatisfaction	43	46	89
Personal reasons	7	6	13
Personal/career futherance	69	52	121
Interest in social/preventive aspects of nursing	94	77	171
Sample size**	183	216	399

* Questionnaire 1 part 1 question 2
** 6 responses missing to marital status question

Table 6

REASONS FOR ENTERING HEALTH VISITING ANALYSED BY MARITAL STATUS *

Content analysis category	MARITAL STATUS		Total
	Single	Married	
Domestic circumstances	31	82	113
Move from hospital or district	13	18	31
Further career or education	120	138	258
Interest in people/health education/preventive medicine	122	131	253
Sample size**	183	216	399

* Questionnaire 1 part 1 question 3
** 6 responses missing to marital status question

Again the responses were content analysed. However, as it was hoped to examine whether the areas of work that provided satisfaction were the same as those that were seen as making a significant contribution, the same categories were used for analysing both.

Tables 7 and 8 show the results of the overall count for the questionnaires. Tutors from the training centres also answered the question on contribution and these results are included. It is obvious that certain areas of work are important to health visitors such as health education and work with mothers and babies/small children. However, it is interesting to note that this latter as such is not accorded importance by the tutors. Differences can be noted between areas of satisfaction and contribution over the period of the research. It was found in the event that there was not a significant association between these two areas. Tables such as these can give the basis for many useful discussions as well as point up areas for further investigation.

These examples illustrate the way in which open-ended questions can be used in questionnaires and their responses reduced to a meaningful and manageable set of categories. Once in this form responses can then be compared, contrasted, linked with other variables and generally manipulated to produce a wealth of useful information and indicators.

B. Likert scale statements

The Likert scale (Likert, 1932) scales attitudes on one, single dimension based on the notion of a quantitative continuum along which people can be arrayed, depending on the magnitude of the attitude which they possess. An important feature of Likert scaling is that the best source of items are the statements typical respondents make when expressing themselves naturally on the topic. Consequently, it is an easier technique to devise than many scalar techniques. Indeed, it appears according to McKennall (1977) to have become the most popular method of attitude scale construction in use today.

Respondents are asked to state the degree to which they endorse or complete the statement made on a five point scale. Several such statements were used to gauge overall response to health visiting and its professional training.

Two examples are given below:

I find health visiting _____.
(very satisfying)/(satisfying)/(neither satisfying nor dissatisfying)/
(dissatisfying)/(very dissatisfying)

Health visiting _____ my expectations.
(greatly exceeds)/(exceeds)/(matches)/(is less than)/(is considerably less than)

Respondents were asked to underline the phrase in each case so that the completed statement most resembled their feelings.

Table 7

GREATEST WELFARE CONTRIBUTION TO THE COMMUNITY*

Content analysis category	Questionnaire number			Tutor
	1	2	3	
Work with particular groups:				
Geriatrics	28	31	30	0
Mothers/babies/preschool children	73	84	85	2
School children/work	1	14	16	1
The handicapped	1	3	6	0
Families	16	42	59	5
Areas of work:				
Health education/preventive medicine	174	154	124	20
Contact with people/giving advice	39	37	32	7
Membership of community team	68	91	69	15
Miscellaneous	15	19	17	0
Total number of responses	415	475	438	50
Sample size	250			26

Questionnaire 1 - Part 3 question 23
Questionnaire 2 - Part 4 question 8
Questionnaire 3 - Part 4 question 6

Table 8

SATISFYING ASPECTS OF THE WORK*

Content analysis category	Questionnaire number 1	2
Work with particular groups:		
Geriatrics	79	76
Mothers/babies/preschool children	130	150
School children/work	11	38
The handicapped	9	15
Families	41	84
Area of work:		
Health education/preventive medicine	121	115
Contact with people/giving advice	61	44
Membership of community team	40	67
Other parts of work:		
Working conditions	1	1
Independence/own initiative	7	7
Miscellaneous	26	30
Total number of responses	526	627
Sample size	250	250

* Questionnaire 1 - Part 3 question 22
  Questionnaire 2 - Part 4 question 7

Tables 9 -12 indicate the responses to these two statements at the end of training and after one year of work. Health visiting certainly appears to receive a very positive evaluation and in direct contrast to the fears being expressed in the profession. For 60% of the sample, these feelings did not apparently change even as a result of their work experience. Further analysis revealed that married health visitors were proportionately more satisfied and had their expectations met more than those who were single.

SATISFACTION WITH HEALTH VISITING* *Table 9*

		Level of Satisfaction					
		1	2	3	4	5	Sample size
Questionnaire number	2	47	124	65	13	1	250
	3	55	122	55	16	2	250

Table 10

		Satisfaction response in questionnaire 2					
		1	2	3	4	5	Sample size
Questionnaire 3	Same response	31	78	32	6	1	148
	Different responses	16	46	33	7	0	102
	Total	47	124	65	13	1	250

$X^2 = 5.8724$ df = 4 $\propto = .05$ p > .05   ∴ Not significant

Satifaction with health visiting — Key to responses

1 - Very satisfying
2 - Satisfying
3 - Neither satisfying nor dissatisfying
4 - Dissatisfying   * Questionnaire 2 part 3 question 13
5 - Very dissatisfying   Questionnaire 3 part 3 question 14

EXPECTATIONS OF HEALTH VISITING* *Table 11*

		Matching of expectations					
		1	2	3	4	5	Sample size
Questionnaire number	2	9	40	158	42	1	250
	3	6	37	154	42	11	250

Table 12

| | | Expectation response in questionnaire 2 | | | | | |
		1	2	3	4	5	Sample size
	Same response	4	23	122	13	1	163
Questionnaire 3	Different response	5	17	36	29	0	87
	Total	9	40	158	42	1	250

$X^2 = 35.0518$ $df = 4$ $\alpha = .05$ $p < .001$ ∴ Highly significant

Expectations of health visiting — Key to responses
1 - greatly exceeds
2 - exceeds
3 - matches
4 - is less than   *Questionnaire 2, part 3, Qu. 14
5 - is considerably less than   Questionnaire 3, part 3, Qu. 15.

Likert scales as mentioned before are easy to construct and are easy to respond to. Because of this they are an important device open to researchers when looking at attitudes. The examples quoted from this research illustrate the ease with which they may be analysed and presented. Obviously, results may be taken much further and sophisticated statistical computations performed. However, they are a tool open for use at both the simple and the sophisticated level and this makes them invaluable.

C. Semantic differential scales

The semantic differential is an attribute sorting technique and is probably the best known of this type. It is a highly generalisable technique of measurement devised by Osgood, Suci and Tannenbaum (1957) and has to be adapted specifically to the requirements of the research problem to which it is applied.

Subjects are asked to tick on a number of scales for a variety of concepts chosen by the researcher as being of relevance to and representative of the area of research interest. The scales are each bi-polar and should be relevant to the concepts. Each scale is assumed to have the property of equal intervals and so may be statistically analysed at a high level.

The concepts in this research were seen as being relevant either to the profession in general or to specific work content or to specific training course content. It was believed that the profiles derived would indicate the perceptions of the sample and would allow a comparison over time that would not be possible in this way with any other technique.

The questionnaires each contained twelve concepts of which eight were repeated throughout all three. Concepts ranged from nursing, health visiting, health education through to sociology. Respondents were asked to rate the words on the basis of what they meant to them. An 'X' was to be placed on each of the scales whereever they felt the word should be rated. Diagram 1 shows one of the questionnaire pages. The need for fast working was emphasised.

The first step in putting this type of information together is to assign the values of the point on the scale to each of the crosses. This then allows the calculation to be made of the average or mean position for all the sample or parts of the sample on each of the scales. From this a profile can be constructed. In diagram 2 profiles for each of the three questionnaires have been drawn for the concept 'health visiting'. The profiles display in an easy visual form both the positions on the various scales including their relation to each other as well as showing immediately the areas of movement over time.

The same scales are used for each concept. This means that reactions to different concepts may be compared. Diagrams 3 and 4 contrast the concepts of nursing and health visiting at the start of the training course and after a year at work. Diagram 5 and 6 show the same for doctor and health visitor. Both of these contrasts of concepts are important in health visiting. The health visitor makes many of her contacts with the community through the doctor. How does she see herself in relation to this person? In what ways does she identify with nursing and yet differentiate herself from this profession? The semantic differential profiles give very quick indications of answers to these questions

Deeper analysis may be made of semantic differential profiles than just visual inspections. Statistical analysis through t-tests for instance may be made of shifts in position. All of the shifts of more than approximately half a position on the scales for the concepts illustrated here were statistically significant. A more sophisticated tool of analysis that can be used is factor analysis. This is a technique that explores the data to see whether some underlying pattern of relationships exists such that the data may be arranged or reduced to a smaller set of 'factors' that may account for the observed interrelations. Child (1970) gives a very good explanation of this technique and its use.

Diagram 1

HEALTH VISITING

Rating

	1	2	3	4	5	6	7 ⇒	
Difficult	:	:	:	:	:	:	:	:	Easy
Progressive	:	:	:	:	:	:	:	:	Traditional
Warm	:	:	:	:	:	:	:	:	Cold
Necessary	:	:	:	:	:	:	:	:	Unnecessary
Hostile	:	:	:	:	:	:	:	:	Friendly
Flexible	:	:	:	:	:	:	:	:	Rigid
Interesting	:	:	:	:	:	:	:	:	Boring
Democratic	:	:	:	:	:	:	:	:	Hierarchical
Satisfying	:	:	:	:	:	:	:	::	Dissatisfying
Harmful	:	:	:	:	:	:	:	:	Beneficial
Organised	:	:	:	:	:	:	:	:	Chaotic
Slow	:	:	:	:	:	:	:	:	Fast

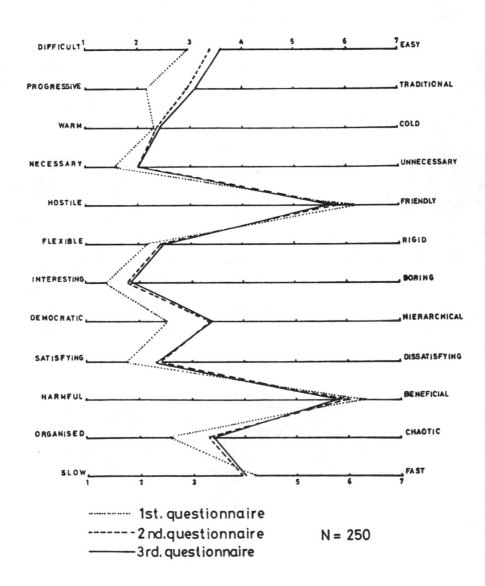

Diagram 2

HEALTH VISITING

Mean score profiles on semantic differential scales for sample answering 3 questionnaires

············· 1st. questionnaire

------- 2nd. questionnaire

———— 3rd. questionnaire

N = 250

Diagram 3

NURSING - HEALTH VISITING

Mean score profiles on semantic differential scales for 1st.questionnaire

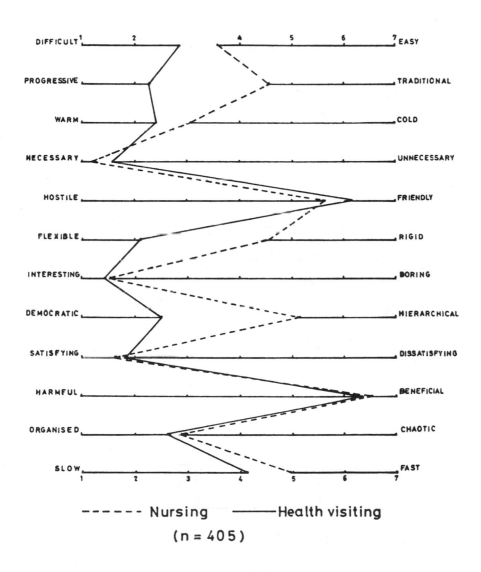

------ Nursing   ———Health visiting

(n = 405)

NURSING – HEALTH VISITING Diagram 4

Mean score profiles on semantic differential scales for 3rd questionnaire

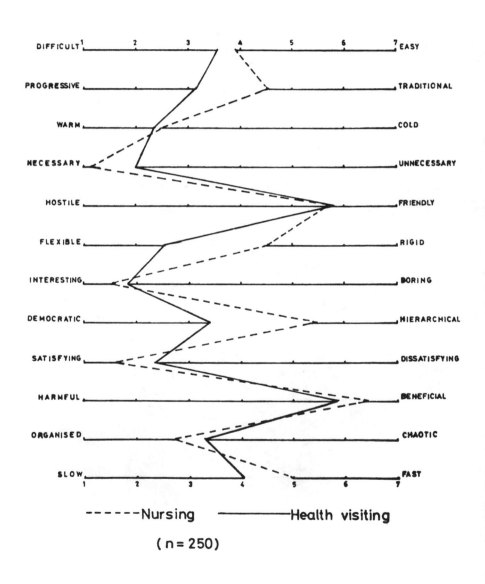

------ Nursing   ——— Health visiting

(n = 250)

Diagram 5

DOCTOR – HEALTH VISITOR

Mean score profiles on semantic differential scales for 1st. questionnaire

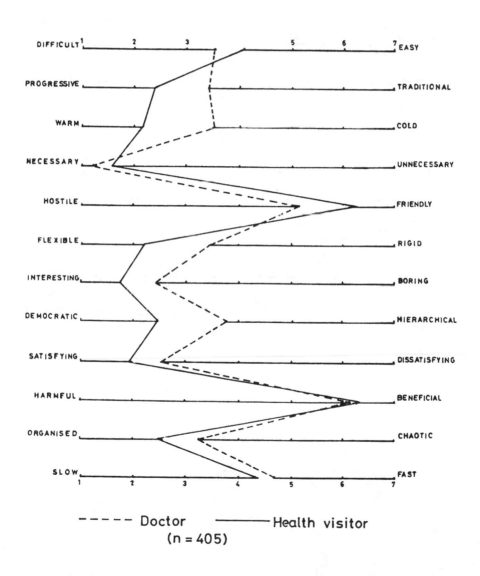

```
- - - - Doctor ———— Health visitor
              (n = 405)
```

Diagram 6

DOCTOR - HEALTH VISITOR

Mean score profiles on semantic differential
scales for 3rd. questionnaire

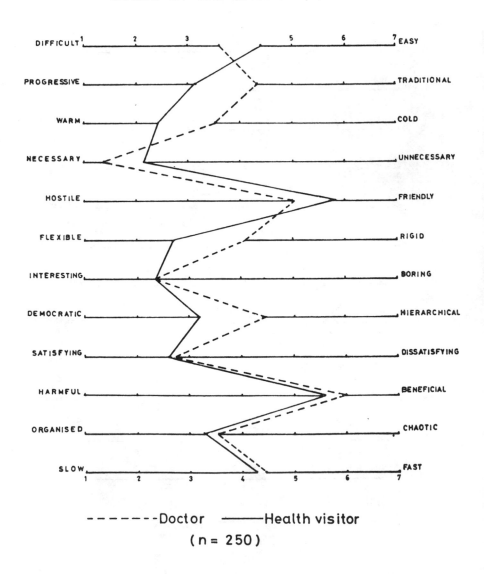

- - - - - - Doctor ————— Health visitor

(n = 250)

Reponses to several of the concepts were factor analysed. Two major factors were found to underlie the pattern of reponses. The one, which could possibly be entitled 'personal stimulation' was composed of the scales satisfying-dissatisfying, interesting-boring, necessary-unnecessary, warm-cold. The other which could be called an 'organisational assessment' factor was made up of the scales flexible-rigid, progressive-traditional, democratic-hierarchical, warm-cold. This second group of scales could all be seen as an evaluation of health visiting or health education in their way of working or organisation as opposed to the first group which is concerned with the personal feelings generated.

Health visitors appear to therefore evaluate their profession and one of its main components for the personal stimulation derived and on the basis of the nature of its organisation. Diagram 2 shows very clearly that there are shifts inward on both 'factors' but particularly for organisational assessment. Are health visitors perhaps expecting a greater degree of flexibility and autonomy than is to be found in the profession? Certainly the pattern is repeated for health education (diagram 7).

Do tutors on training courses perhaps influence their new entrants in their perception of the profession? The semantic differential profile for tutors for health education does not appear to replicate that of their students either at the start or end of the course (diagram 8) although there are some important points of similarity. However, it would appear that the geographical area of training may have some influence on attitudes such as that towards health education (diagram 9). Differences between the North of England & London & South East were often statistically significant.

It may be that the use of the semantic differential opens up more questions than it answers. Undoubtedly it provides a multidimensional view in a way that no other technique does and therefore the potential for use is enormous. Obviously this is not a technique that can easily be coped with on any scale without recourse to a computer especially for factor analysis. For those fortunate enough to have access then the S.P.S.S. (Statistical Package for the Social Sciences) computer package is the most convenient answer. It is easier if there are some helpful experts around to guide the novice through her first experience of it.

4. Basic Decisions : Contraints on Data Collection

There are many benefits to be derived from the use of questionnaires as a research tool as outlined at the start of section 3 and they may be constructed apparently with ease. Consequently questionnaires are often long and samples large as the researcher gets carried away with the possibilities opened up by this method.

Diagram 7

HEALTH EDUCATION

Mean score profiles on semantic differential scales for sample answering 3 questionnaires

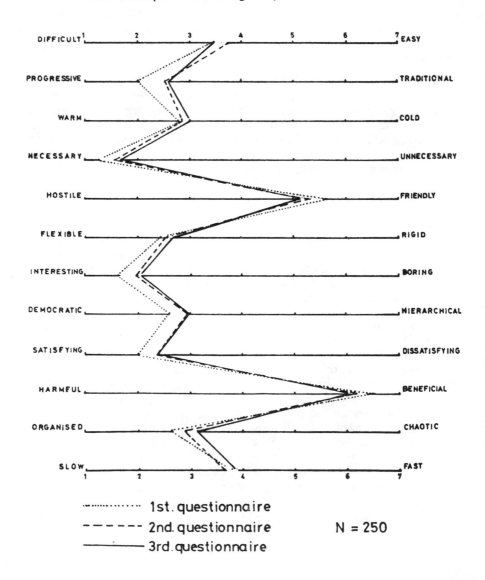

············· 1st. questionnaire

－ － － － － 2nd. questionnaire   N = 250

————— 3rd. questionnaire

Diagram 8

HEALTH EDUCATION

Mean score profiles on semantic differential scales for tutors and students

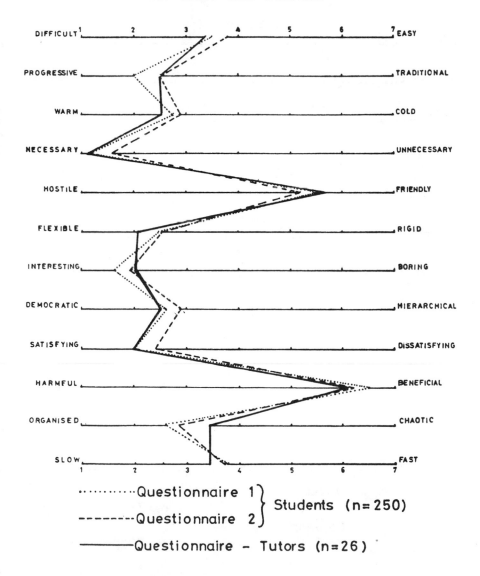

·········· Questionnaire 1 ⎫
                          ⎬ Students (n=250)
-------- Questionnaire 2 ⎭

———— Questionnaire – Tutors (n=26)

Diagram 9

HEALTH EDUCATION

Mean score profiles on semantic differential scales for 2nd. questionnaire

BY REGION

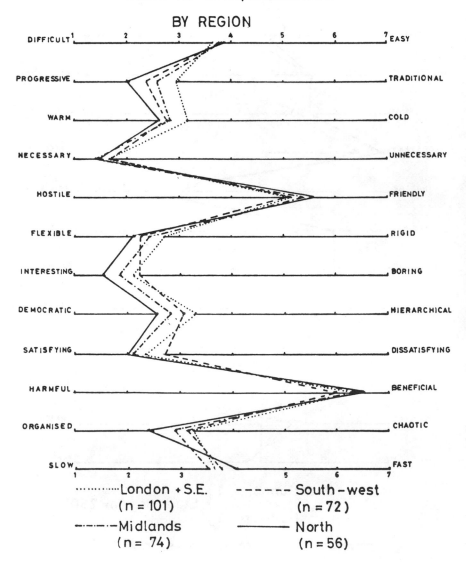

Length of questionnaire is not a factor that necessarily affects response rates (Scott, 1961). However, it is important that a compromise is sought between asking questions on all the areas of interest to the researcher and at the same time retaining the interest and motivation of the respondent. The use of several different techniques such as those illustrated may well serve to maintain this interest as well as widening the picture for the researcher.

Another important consideration that needs an early decison is on the type or types of analysis to be carried out. Time and labour may both be constraining factors. Computers can often alleviate some of these constraints but they also can introduce many other problems. Unless analysis is thought out carefully at an early stage the scope of the problem can be overwhelming when the answered questionnares return.

100 people answering 10 questions produce 1,999 total replies each of which may be extensive depending on the nature of the questions. 200 people and 20 questions produce 4,000 replies; so the numbers rapidly increase. From this it is obvious that two crucial decisions have to be made early on - the number and type of questions to be used and the size of the sample. There is no easy formula or set answer for these decisions.

Sample size
In determining the sample size it can be useful to consider the following questions:

-   are there characteristics that need to be met within the sample?
-   if there are comparisons to be made over time, what allowance needs to be made for attrition ie. sample drop-out?
-   what administrative constraints exist within the study?
-   what analytical tools/manpower are available?

The answers to these questions in the health visitor study were important in determining the structure and size of the overall sample.

It was decided that two characteristics should be present in the sample as it was felt that they might be important. These were geographical location and educational category of training establishment. To facilitate the drawing up of a sample to reflect these characteristics, a two-way grid was laid out with the four major geographical regions on one axis and the four main categories of training establishment on the other. This gave a grid with 16 cells. Colleges were then allocated to the relevant cell. It was decided that 50% of new entrants that particular year should be contacted in order to allow for sample attrition over the course of the research. Administrative constraints made it easier to sample whole training courses rather than take a sample of students from each. The relevant number and distribution of colleges was easily decided in the light of these needs and constraints.

A decision to use postal questionnaires was determined mainly by administrative constraints rather than methodological considerations. There was only one researcher full time with a sample spread over England and Wales and the need to contact them all within the space of two weeks to ensure that all the responses were from the same stage of training and work. Luckily the cost of postage could be lost in the organisational spending and so this aspect of budgetting was not a problem.

Conclusion

If questionnaires are seen to be the most appropriate tool for a piece of research then many decisions will have to be taken as a result of this. These will cover the nature of the questionnaire, including its length and layout, administration and analysis and the size and structure of the sample. The decisions are not independent of each other but very interralated. The needs of the research and the researcher will often constrain the scope of the study.

In this chapter, it is hoped that the description of various questioning techniques and their illustration from a large scale study within health visiting itself will perhaps provide some ideas that will be useful to health visitors faced with this sort of decision making.

BIBLIOGRAPHY

Anderson, E.R. (1973), *The Role of the Nurse,* Royal College of Nursing, London.
Child, D. (1070), *The Essentials of Factor Analysis*, Holt, Rinehart & Winston, London.
Ellis, P. (1980), *Job Satisfaction amongst Health Visitors*, Ph.D. Thesis, University of Bradford.
Jameson Report, (1956), *An Enquiry into Health Visiting*, Ministry of Health, Dept. of health Scotland and Dept. of Education, HMSO, London.
Likert, R. (1932), "A technique for the measurement of attitudes", *Archives of Psychology*, No. 140, New York.
Locke, E.A. (1976) "The nature and causes of job satisfaction" in Dunnette M.D. (ed.), *Handbook of Industrial and Organisational Psychology*, Rand McNally College Publishing Company, Chicago.
MacGuire, J. (1966), *From Student to Nurse*, Oxford Area Nurse Training Committee, Oxford.
McKennell, A.C. (1977), "Attitude scale construction" in O'Muircheartaigh, C.A. & Payne, C. (eds.), *The Analysis of Survey Data*, Vol 1, *Exploring Data Structures*, John Wiley, London.

O'Muircheartaigh, C.A., (1977), "Statistical analysis in the context of survey research", in O'Muircheartaigh, C.A. & Payne, C. (eds.), *The Analysis of Survey Data*, Vol. 1, *Exploring Data Structures*, John Wiley, London.

Osgood, C.E., Suci, G.J. & Tannenbaum, P.H. (1957), *The Measurement of Meaning*, Univ. of Illinios Press, Urbana, Illinois.

Scott, C. (1961), "Research on mail surveys", *Journal of the Royal Statistical Society. A.,* *124,* 143-195.

Singh, A. (1970), *The Student Nurse on Experimental Courses, Part 1: Attitude towards Nursing as a Career,* General Nursing Council for England & Wales, London.

Chapter 7

An Enquiry into Child Health Surveillance
Procedures undertaken by Health Visitors in England*

Phil Connolly

This study set out to identify child health policies involving health visitors and to find out health visitors' views of their work with children. The objectives were, first, to survey health visiting historically to find out how the work developed in dealing with children; second to identify differences in child health policies and assess their influence on the work of health visitors; and third, to explore the realms of health visiting practice and attempt to identify features which health visitors hold in common and might be termed 'practice theories'.

The main findings are summarised and discussed briefly below. The historical survey showed that the work of health visitors in many respects has changed little over the last 150 years. At the turn of this century health visitors worked mainly with the poorest sector of the population but at the present time they are part of a state national health scheme dealing with all ages and sectors of the population. While the scope of work has widened for health visitors the findings in this study show that the role is mainly still in health teaching and most of the work is in dealing with young children.

Study Methods

The investigation is based on two sources of data. One source obtained from a postal enquiry of 90 Area Health Authorities (AHAs). Eighty eight authorities responded and provided a plethora of data on their child health policies and health visitor involvement in this work. The other source of data was obtained from a convenience sample of 34 health visitors selected from 12 health districts in one regional health authority in the south of England.

Part One

Area Health Authority Child Health Policies

Many AHAs' replies used the terms 'assessment', 'developmental

*Based on a thesis submitted for M.Phil. to Polytechnic of North London.

assessment', and 'screening procedures', interchangeably Hearing tests were referred to specifically. In the analysis these terms are categorised together and regarded as situations which involved health visitors in implementing these aspects of child care policies. Three types of policy and health visitor involvement were identified:

1. 'Non-specified assessment' policy (19 AHAs). Health visitors were not required to assess childrens' development but twelve of the 19 AHAs required them to carry out hearing tests. In seven of the 19 AHAs only doctors were responsible for developmental assessments on children. This 'non specified assessment' situation was under review in four of the 19 AHAs.

2. 'General assessment' policy (15 AHAs). Health visitors were expected to assess childrens' development. The assessment procedure was discretionary but guidelines were issued by AHAs for health visitors to use in this work. In six of the 15 AHAs health visitors carried out hearing tests on children. Doctors or health visitors assessed childrens' development in the 15 AHAs. The assessment situation depended on opportune contact with children, more than the expertise of the assessor.

3. 'Specified assessment' policy (54 AHAs). Developmental assessment programmes were organised, both doctors and health visitors participated in this work. Assessments on children were carried out by health visitors and doctors at ages specified by the AHA. Record forms linked with the assessment procedure, and printed on these forms were the specific assessment age, number of assessments, and assessment criteria associated with each age. All health visitors carried out hearing tests.

The findings of a survey of health visitors and hearing tests by the Health Visitors' Association (1978)[1] were similar to those of this study. For example, the HVA found health visitors in 87% of health districts tested childrens' hearing compared with 82% in this study of health authorities. One of the AHAs in this study in their reply stated that a valid hearing test did not exist and in this Area health visitors only tested childrens' hearing for high frequency loss. As so many health visitors are testing childrens' hearing, more information is needed to find out which tests they are carrying out, how effective these tests are in identifying hearing defects, and how health visitors are trained in these techniques.

In the 15 'general assessment' policy AHAs the health visitors are issued with guidelines or schedules to assist them in this work. These included five Sheridan guides (1975)[2], two Denver Tests (1968)[3], one Griffiths Scale

(1970)[4], and seven schedules devised by AHA working parties consisting of health visitors and nurse managers.

The record forms of 54 'specified assessment' policy AHAs showed the ages at assessment, and number and frequency of assessments required to be carried out by health visitors on children in the first year of life and over the first five years of life (Table 1). In the main the number of assessments were minimal in the first year and increased in the following years.

Table [1]

Number of AHAs 'specified assessments' by health visitors during the first year of life and over the first five years.

Number of assessments	AHAs expected assessments in first year of life. N = 54	AHAs expected assessments over first five years of life. N = 54
0	5	
1	4	1
2	12	6
3	24	7
4	6	12
5	3	5
6		10
7		8
8		3
9		2

Four peak assessment ages were identified, (figure 1), at six weeks (28 AHAs), 6 months (31 AHAs), eighteen months (33 AHAs) and 3 years (34 AHAs).

None of the AHAs record forms contained scales or grading schemes to allow for individual differences in children or in their developmental progress. Many forms required definitive pass/fail, positive/negative results, for example in regard to hearing and vision testing. Printed on the record forms were criteria associated with aspects of child development that AHAs required health visitors to assess. The findings (Table 2) show little agreement amongst AHAs on these assessment criteria.

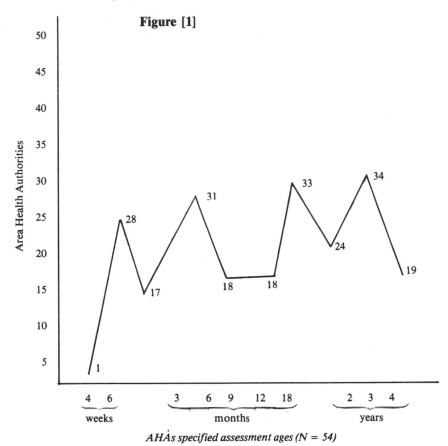

AHAs specified assessment ages (N = 54)

A feature constant in the findings was the 'instrumental directive' nature of child health records. In this study, the term 'instrumental directives' is applied to records which are tools with the potential to influence child care work in general and health visiting work in particular. The employers of health visitors use records to control aspects of health visiting work, for example, the AHAs who provide records on which are prescribed childrens' developmental assessment ages, number of assessments and developmental criteria to be assessed. Legally health visitors records provide evidence of work they have done or failed to do. These records also can convey concerns of health visitors in cases of child neglect and abuse. For health visitors, their records can be one means of demonstrating competance in work as most aspects of work are difficult to monitor.

Table [2]   AHA assessment criteria printed on record
forms at four peak assessment ages.

Assessment Criteria	Assessment Ages			
	6 weeks N = 28	6 months N = 31	18 months N = 33	3 years N = 34
General Appearance				
Health	5	1	1	5
Hips	8			
Height	8	6	1	
Weight	5	6	1	
Head Circumference	7	3		
Gender	2			
Nutrition State	3			
Fontanelles	1		1	
Teeth				14
Vision				
Follows Mother	11			
Dangling Object	6			
Turns to Light	6			
Reacts to moving person	2			
Fixates on object 10^{II} away	13			
Follows object or person		19		
Squint		9	14	19
Watches distance away			6	
Stycar Test				22
Colour Matching				14
Hearing and Speech				
Hearing Test	11	21	6	22
Smile response to sound	4			
Cooing	13			
Inhibition to sound 6^{II}	9			
Responds to mothers voice	11			
Startles	4			
Vocalises		29		
Uses number of words			29	
Obeys commands		22		
Sentences				18
Communication and words				25
Motor Activity				
Stepping	6			
Grasp	11			
Head Lag	17			
Ventral Suspension	22			

Cont...

Table 2 *Cont.*

Assessment Criteria	Assessment Ages			
	6 weeks N = 28	6 months N = 31	18 months N = 33	3 years N = 34
Motor Activity (Continued)				
Fisting	8			
Pelvis high/low	7			
Primary back curve	3			
Symmetrical movements	8			
Sits with support		31		
Bears weight		27		
Head control		16		
Grasp		19		
Transfers objects/each hand		21		
Reaches		22		
Chews food		5		
Hand control			30	
Crawls			3	
Runs, walks, climbs			33	
Draws				28
Balances				30
Large body movements				17
Builds tower with cubes				25
Social Interaction				
Smile response to voice	15			
Smiles not to contact	15			
Response to voice	7			
Stops crying when given attention	10			
Follows human face	3			
Vocalises in response to voice		15		
Listens interprets situ.		7		
Feeds self			19	12
Dresses self			8	18
Toilet trained			16	22
Plays with other children				11

As health visitors' child health records have the potential to contain a rich source of data on the health status of children nationally, as such they are an important resource tool. They can help identify health trends and influence or support child health policies. The findings in this study show that considerable variation exists in health visitors child health recording schemes for the under five age group. There is an urgent need to review the situation and introduce an efficient national record for monitoring childrens' progress and which will contribute to a national child health surveillance programme.

Part Two

Health Visitors' Views of their Child Care Work

This part of the study examines health visitors' views of their work with children. The objectives were fourfold; first, to find out views on child health policies; second, to examine 'health' as a measureable entity in health visiting practice; third, to identify characteristics which might be termed 'operational knowledge' in the realms of health visiting; and fourth, to examine autonomy and professionalisation in health visiting.

In terms of professional socialisation where an individual goes through the process of internalising the norms, values and knowledge of the professional group, health visitor students are required to undergo an enormous amount of personal change in a short time. The weighting of the subject matter on the course is on the academic side. Because of the limited time available for practical training it means that tutors to the course rely heavily on background experiences of students on which to build health visiting skills.

The health visitor sample had a variety of midwifery experience prior to their health visitor training, table (3).

Table [3]   Midwifery experience prior
to health visitor training;

Midwifery Course	Health Visitors N = 34
State Certified Midwife (SCM)	15
Central Midwives Board (Pt 1)	4
Obstetric Course (12 weeks)	15

Differences were observed in the way health visitors valued their nursing backgrounds as a pre-requisite requirement for health visiting work. Nineteen health visitors thought this experience was very useful, ten, only fairly useful and five not useful in any way. Two of the latter undertook nurse training only to become health visitors.

Child Health Policies and Health Visiting Practice
Of the thirty four health visitors 20 worked in 'specified assessment' policy AHAs and 14 worked in 'non-specified assessment' policy AHAs. A

comparison was made between the AHAs specified assessment ages (54) and the assessment ages preferred by health visitors (34), Table (4).

Table (4) Assessment ages recommended by health visitors and AHAs

Assessment Ages	N = 34	%	AHAs N = 34	%
2 weeks	4	12	0	0
4 weeks	7	20	1	2
6 weeks	10	18	28	52
3 months	13	38	17	31
6 months	23	68	31	57
7 months	5	15	0	0
8 months	4	12	0	0
9 months	7	20	18	33
12 months	15	44	18	33
18 months	22	65	33	61
2 years	26	76	24	44
3 years	16	48	34	63
4 years	17	50	19	29

An analysis was made of health visitors' home visiting programmes to look at some of the issues which led to these visits. The findings are based on visits which health visitors made on the morning prior to their interview. Table (5) lists the types of visits undertaken and shows a considerable amount of time involved in advisory visits. Problem centred visits outweighted other visits, but, for at least half, the health visitor routine visits were a reality. Seven of the 20 health visitors who worked in 'specified assessment' policy AHAs carried out developmental assessments and notably, no specific assessments were carried out by health visitors in 'non-specified assessment' policy AHAs but some assessment was carried out on the 11 assessed children with developmental problems (Table 5, b).

Table (5) Home Visits made by health visitors on one morning:

Type of home visit	Health visitors N = 34
(a) *Advisory visits*	
New births	34
New families in the area	24
Routine visits to under 5s	19
Developmental assessments	7
(b) *Problem centred visits*	
Child development problems	11

Cont.

Table 5 *Cont.*

Type of home visit	Health visitors N = 34
(b) *Problem centred visits* (*Continued*)	
Support visits	11
·Crisis visits	19
Families with multiple problems	4
Sick children	5
Non-accidental injury cases	2
Follow up previous problem	2
(c) *Liaison visits*	
Hospital follow up	7
G.P. referrals	6
Housing reports	6
(d) *Promoting health policies*	
Encouraging immunisation	8
Non-clinic attendance	6

Note: More than one type of visit made by some health visitors.

The health visitor's case loads in this study ranged from 150 - 500 families which means that for those with large numbers, time is an important consideration when assessing 'health'. Lawrence and Skarloff (1978)[5] found little difference in the time health visitors and doctors took to assess childrens' development (mean time 18.4 minutes if under one year of age). The health visitors in this study took a mean time of 15.9 minutes to assess a child. Differences were observed in assessment time of health visitors in 'specified assessment' policy AHAs and 'non specified assessment' policy AHAs. The former took longer (mean time 16 minutes) than the latter (mean time 15 minutes).

The findings (figure 2) show the amount of time health visitors spent in dealing with feeding, behaviour, child development, safety, sleep and skin care. Ninety seven per cent of the health visitors spent a lot of time in discussions dealing with feeding. This was followed closely by time involved with behaviour problems, developmental assessments and sleep issues which took up 68% of time. In regard to child assessment policies it appears that in spite of the AHA policy, 14 of the health visitors in 'non specified assessment' policy AHAs still spent a lot of their time assessing children's development.

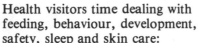

Health visitors time dealing with
feeding, behaviour, development,
safety, sleep and skin care:

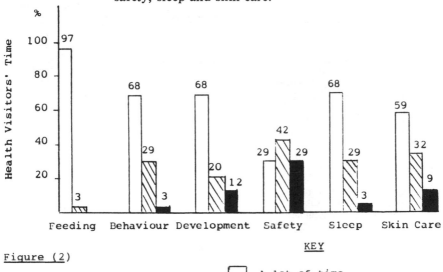

Figure (2)

KEY

☐ A lot of time

▨ Not too much time

■ Very little time

Practice Theory

Bishop (1978)[6] defines reality in the work situation as 'the application of operational knowledge'. In Berger and Luckman's (1966)[7] terms the practitioner's sense of reality and comprehension of and certainty about events and objects presented, is his or her knowledge in a particular realm. According to Luker (1978)[8] some health visitors believe their work is too subtle or intangible to be assessed. If this was true, no one, including clients, would be aware of the health visitors' effect and there would hardly be a reason for continuing to practice. The limitations of the study resources enabled only an exploratory study to be undertaken of 'operational knowledge' in the realm of health visiting work. With children it was hoped that the findings would provide a framework on which further research might be undertaken later.

The health visitors were asked 'what do you look for when assessing a child in the home?' In Table (6) are listed the unedited responses to this question.

Table (6)   What do you look for when assessing a child?

Observation	Number of Health Visitors
Home environment: Excessive dirt, neglect unsafe:	34
Expression on child's face	34
Crying (reason or cause)	32
Relationship between mother and child (child clinging to mother)	29
Reaction of child to strangers (if friendly and alert)	28
Deviations in milestone development	21
Mothers reaction to visit (HVs)	16
Physical condition of child (as presented)	16
Child's size, height, weight (related to parents size)	15
Condition of child's hair and skin (spots, blemishes or bruises)	15
Palor and signs of illness	11
Nutritional state (over/under weight, on correct diet)	11
Mother's interest in child's physical and emotional needs (way she talks about child's care; questions she asks and way she reacts herself to questions on child	11
Appearance of child (subdued, withdrawn, fidgets)	9
Child's ability to communicate verbally	9
Type of clothing worn by child (appropriate for weather, size and growth)	6
Father and mothers attitude (ambivalent, over protective)	6
Sleep habits of child and household (regular or erratic sleep pattern)	6
Child always asleep (when HV visits)	3
Excessive discipline (parents realistic or unrealistic expectations)	3
Relationship between child and other siblings	3
Eyes (bright, clear, squint)	3
House proud mother, over tidy home (over anxious)	2
Toys provided for child and opportunities to explore environment	2
Sex of the child (and is this the child intended (HV) to see)	2
Number and condition of child's teeth	2
Clean or dirty child	1

The above findings show that health visitors do not always agree on assessment criteria. One reason for this lack of agreement may be due to the problem of defining 'normality' in children. This is not surprising when leading experts on children do not always agree on this subject. Three assessment criteria mentioned most frequently by the health visitors were - 'physical environment of the home which might harm the child' (34), 'expression on a child's face' (34) and 'distressed crying' (32). The 'expression' criterion was frequently qualified by the health visitors as 'a look of happiness', 'anxiety', 'apathy' or 'withdrawal'. The mother child relationship was judged by twenty-nine health visitors by 'their feeling', 'impression' or 'intuition'.

Sixteen health visitors said the mother's reaction to their visit influenced the time they stayed and this reflected what they were able to observe about the child and the home situation. One health visitor who worked in a deprived inner city area found first visits very difficult as people thought she came to inspect their homes. This health visitor introduced herself as 'from the welfare' and explained her role later when the family knew her better. Confusion over the clients' understanding of the health visitors' role is well documented (Newson J. and Newson E. 1965[9]; Land H. 1969[10]; Hunt M. 1972[11]; Clark J. 1973[12]; Wilson H. & Herbert C. 1978[13]).

The assessment criteria listed by the 34 health visitors (table 6) were compared with the assessment criteria on the AHA record forms (table 2). The findings showed that the health visitors extended their observations of children beyond those required on the AHA record forms. Twenty one health visitors looked for 'deviations in milestone development' and none mentioned that this feature linked with the health authority child developmental assessment policy or record form assessment requirements. Only the criteria 'height' 'weight' 'nutrition' 'gender' 'vision' 'hearing' and 'fontanelles' appear on both table (2) and table (6). The assessment criteria listed by the health visitors provide 'ingredients' for a 'child health' assessment model. With further sifting, interpretation, discussion and research these assessment criteria could contribute to the formation of a comprehensive 'child care model' for interdisciplinary workers' use.

Ranson (1977)[14] argues that health visitors should stop cultivating a professional image and stop acting like second class doctors. The findings in table (6) did not confirm this medical tendency. The language the health visitors used to describe their observations on children was that used in every day life. It is argued in this study that because these observations concern human every day life they must necessarily be expressed in the language of the society in which the observers and observed live. What is at issue is the health visitors' claim for professional recognition. The concepts and purpose of what they are doing in society, need to be implicitly and explicitly defined in ways which they and others understand, as there is a dearth of data on these issues at the present time.

Health Visiting and Professionalisation

Wilensky's (1964)[15] developmental sequence in professionalisation provides one way of viewing health visiting as a profession. He sets out stages along a continuum which starts with a new practice recruited from other occupations; training facilities which lead to standards and recognition; the development of a professional association, and political agitation to gain support for territory and an ethical code. At the end of the last century, doctors, teachers and sanitary inspectors brought their skills to health visiting work; health visitor training began in 1908 at the Royal Sanitary Institute; one of the earliest professional associations for health visitors was established in 1896, the Women Public Health Officers' Association, now the Health Visitors' Association; and in 1979 health visitors collectively campaigned to ensure their status was recognised in the Nurses, Midwives and Health Visitors Act of 1979.

An underlying issue in this study is concerned with who controls health visiting and this links closely with the concept of autonomy which is central to the notion of professionalism. Etzioni (1969)[16] holds that the essence of professionalism is that it is free from social pressures and free to innovate, experiment and take risks without failure. Whether health visitors are truly independent practitioners is questionable if one looks at the nurse management hierarchy at district and area levels in the National Health Service. Whether health visitors achieve parity with medical practitioners is also arguable and widely discussed (McIntosh and Dingwall (1976)[17], Brooks (1978)[18] and Manson (1977)[19]).

Lortie's (1969)[20] study of teachers provides a basis for looking at autonomy in health visiting work as ther are some similarities in both teachers' and health visitors' work situations. Lortie identified reward systems consisting of extrinsic, ancillary and intrinsic rewards which enable teachers to have some control over their work. Extrinsic rewards represent salary grades, responsibility payments for additional qualifications which teachers receive but not health visitors. Employers of teachers and health visitors offer extrinsic rewards in terms of opportunities for further education by funding courses and granting exemption from work responsibilities whilst studying. These rewards can be a means of controlling staff who are waiting for these opportunities. But once additional qualifications or expertise is acquired, staff in turn can then use these to bargain for changes in work conditions or seek better situations elsewhere. Table (7) sets out the educational opportunities health visitors in this study had taken since their health visitor training.

Ancillary rewards tempt people into an occupation, e.g. hours, holidays, work conditions etc. Health visiting hours like teaching hours are conducive to those with family commitments as most evenings and weekends are free. All but four of the health visitors were married and figures from the CETHV (1980)[21] show that the percentage of married health visitors ranges from 55-75% depending on the area in which they are employed. Generally the percentage is lower in rural areas. The problem according to Lortie is that the attraction of ancillary rewards fades when people witness everyone receiving these benefits as part of every day work

Table (7)   Courses undertaken by health visitors post health visitor training:

Type of Course	Health Visitors N = 34
1. *In-Service Courses*	
Audiology	7
Child development	5
Counselling	4
Sickle/Cell anaemia	2
Crisis intervention & NAI	4
Violence in the family	6
Child psychiatry	1
Spina bifida	1
Mothercraft	1
Dental care	1
Nutrition	1
Dermatology	1
2. *Special Courses*	
Health visitor refresher course	4
Fieldwork teacher course	2
Family planning	3
Relaxation classes	3
Management	1
3. *Courses in Own Time*	
Diploma social science	2
Counselling	1
Pre-school play group	1
Saturday seminars in children's hospital	1
Open university	1
4. *No courses*	10

Note: Some health visitors undertook more than one course.

life. Research is needed to find out if ancillary rewards are a major factor in attracting people into health visiting.

Intrinsic rewards are more difficult to measure but provide some means by which individuals control their work situation. In teaching, teachers are likely to resist interference by administrators or colleagues. Lortie said 'students deny or grant responses which teachers consider as 'payments'.' Health visitors are in a similar situation and 'payment' depends on clients' acceptance or rejection of them, their advice or even their visit. While both teachers and health visitors resist controls over their work at times both need help and advice. The means by which health visitors in this study were provided with opportunities to discuss work problems are listed in table (8) below. Three health visitors (8.8%) had weekly meetings with nursing officers. This compares with 9.8% of teachers in Lortie's study who had similar meetings with heads of departments.

Table (8) Opportunities provided in health districts for health visitors to discuss their work.

Type of meeting	Health Visitors N = 34
Daily contact with colleagues	17
Weekly meetings with nursing officers (informal)	3
Monthly meetings with senior nurse managers (formal)	12
No provision	2

The subject of work satisfaction was explored briefly to find out if this related to autonomy in health visitors' work. Nearly a third (12) of the health visitors were very satisfied with the work they were doing in child care. The frequent comments expressed reflected good work conditions, freedom to develop ideas, and great variety and scope of work. Many (20) of the health visitors were only fairly satisfied and their responses included comments on aspects of work which they felt could be improved. Two health visitors were extremely dissatisfied, mainly because of the lack of opportunities they had to develop ideas and because much of their work involved dealing with family crises.

To summarise the findings of the second part of this study, health visiting as an occupation demonstrates some of the characteristics associated with long standing professions for example medicine, and of other occupations striving to achieve professional status such as teaching. In terms of professional characteristics, health visiting is a young profession. The findings show that health authorities control aspects of health visiting work in varying degrees and this is seen in their child health surveillance policies. The health visitors in this study have considerable potential control over their work particularly in the way they organise their home visiting programmes and in the advice they offer parents during these visits. The findings do suggest that health visitors themselves are not all fully confident in controlling aspects of their work, as over half of the health visitors in this study fatalistically accepted unhappy work situations which they felt were beyond their control. In the health visiting practice situation the findings showed, that regardless of the AHA child health assessment policy, health visitors made their own evaluations of childrens' well-being. This study has only revealed some ideas on 'operational knowledge' which might be termed pragmatic knowledge in defining health in children. There is a need for further research in decision making and the element of risk in the assessment of child health, and the development of health visiting as a profession in that area.

Conclusions and Recommendations

Health visitors on their training course are prepared for health visiting work in general, not in particular. They are taught to refer problems to a variety of specialists. The findings in this study suggest that if developmental assessments are essential for the benefit of all children and if doctors have the required expertise, as indicated in the replies of seven AHAs and supported widely by experts on the subject, then health visitors should stop carrying out work for which they are unqualified. If developmental assessments are in the realm of health visiting and there is a good case for argument as health visitors are already employed to visit homes of children to advise on any difficulty or interruption in their progress, then the findings in this study point to a need to clarify the situation. For example, there is a need to be clear about which aspects of children's development health visitors essentially need to assess; which ages are best at which to assess children's development nationally; what are the minimal number of assessments that need to be made to avoid unneccessary scrutiny; and where in developmental assessment work are health visitors most likely to serve the interests of children in preventing morbidity and mortality.

Because health visiting is a young profession it still has many unclear work boundaries which reflect the diverse use of skills and wide interpretation of the role. This study has only begun to explore one dimension of health visiting work, the work concerning the health of children. There are many other possible fields of study. The nature of the work is such that the health visitors cannot develop people.

People can only develop themselves. Health visitors provide 'anticipatory guidance' to help people take decisions about themselves. This 'anticipatory guidance' is the essence of health visiting but much more research is vital for the development of this subject. Recommendations arising from this study are divided into three areas; management, education, and practice.

Management

Health visitors' immediate nurse managers should be qualified health visitors.

Working parties under the auspices of the CETHV or the new Health Visiting Joint Committee should be set up in each region to examine the health visitors work in child assessment to identify where they can most effectively contribute in this work.

A national health visitor child health record should include:

a. layout that enables forms to be folded to adapt to existing filing cabinets e.g. size A4, A5, and A6.
d. divisions on the forms whereby results of developmental assessments, screening procedures and subjective assessments should be clearly distinguishable.
c. space for parents or those caring for children to comment on the child's progress or needs.

Education

Opportunities should be provided for health visitors to specialise in developmental assessments and screening procedures. The fieldwork teacher with this expertise is in an ideal position to extend her role in this area because of her teacher/manager status and practice work base.

Practice

Health visiting practice research units should be established in the field to encourage and develop research in the practice of health visiting.

Bibliography

1. Health Visitors' Association (1978) *'Survey on Hearing Testing'* Health Visitor, May 1978, Vol *51*.
2. Sheridan M. (1975) *'Children's Developmental Progress'*, NFER
3. *Denver Developmental Scale* (1968) Frankenberg & Doods.
4. Griffiths R. (1970) *'The Abilities of Babies'* Young & Son.
5. Lawrence W. & Sklaroff S.A. (1978) *'Who should carry out developmental screening'* Health Bulletin Vol *36*.
6. Bishop James M. (1978) *'Institutional Knowledge & Operational Knowledge in Work'* Sociology of Occupations Vol 6 Aug 1978 pp328-332.
7. Berger P. & Luckman T. (1966) *The Social Construction of Reality*. London Penguin.
8. Luker Karen A. (1978) *'Goal attainment'* Nursing Times, July 1978.

9. Newson J. & Newson E. (1965) *'Patterns of Infant Care in an Urban community'*. London Allen & Unwin.
10. Land H. (1969) *Large Families in London*. Bell
11. Hunt M. (1972) *The delemma of identity in health visiting*. Nursing Times (Occasional Papers *68* No. 5 17-20 No. 6. 23-24.
12. Clark J. (1973) *A Family Visitor*. Royal College of Nursing.
13. Wilson H. & Herbert C. (1978) *Parents & Children in the Inner City*. London, Routledge and Kegan Paul.
14. Ranson B. (1977) *'The Personal Touch or Professional Image'* Health Visitor Aug. 1977 Vol *50*.
15 Wilensky H. (1964) in Etsionni A. (Ed) (1969) *The Semi Professions & their Organisations*; New York.
16. Etsionni A. (1969) *The Semi Professions & their Organisations*. The Free Press. MacMillan Co.
17. McIntosh J. & Dingwall R. (1976) *Teamwork in theory & practice*. Mimeo. University of Aberdeen.
18. Brooks M. (1973) *Management of the Team in general practice*. Journal of Royal College of General Practitioners *23* 239.
19. Manson T. (1977) *Management, the Professions & the Unions*. In Stacey M. et al (eds) Health and the division of labour. London, Croom Helm.
20. Lortie Dan C. (1969) *'The balance of control and autonomy in elementary school teaching'* in Etsionni A. (1969) The Semi Professions & their Organisations. The Free Press. MacMillan Co.
21. *Manpower Survey, Base Line Report*. CETHV (1980)

Chapter 8

What is the Health Visitor doing in Europe?*

C. Thelma Wilson

Ideas of positive health in Europe and in particular the delivery of the service through the work of the health visitor/public health nurse, are central to the theme of this paper.

The title 'Health Visitor' is not in common usage in the countries of Europe, other than in the U.K., and this has led to confusion as to whether such staff exist elsewhere. The 'Study on Legislation Concerning Nursing Services and education' undertaken by Dr. J. Moerloose for WHO in 1979 states that "within the wealth of nursing specialities community nursing (health visitor, district nurse) is rather uncommon or at least a comparatively rare speciality." Despite this statement, fifteen of the twenty-five European countries in this study had data on 'public health nurses', health studies were sometimes included in the basic nurse education, though more often being a specific post-basic course[1].

At a time when national and internationl bodies have stated policies on the prevention of ill-health and the maintenance of health, the education programme designed for the community nursing staffs have not kept up with the technological sophistication in the courses for curative nurses.

"The fundamental responsibility of the nurse is three-fold; to conserve life, to alleviate suffering and to promote health" (From the International Code of Nursing Ethics adopted by the International Council of Nurses 1953, revised 1965)[2]. The term 'nurse' has been defined variously in law in the European countries and her role and function, as defined, are protected and prescribed. There does not appear to have been the same attention given to the title, role and function of the health visitor/public health nurse.

"Primary health care is the key to achieving an acceptable level of health throughout the world in the forseeable future as part of the social development and in the spirit of social justice"[3]. The nurse is an essential member of the Primary Health Care Team and plays an equal part, with the

100

other members, in striving after 'health' for the people in her charge.

"Article 57(1) of the Treaty establishing the European Economic Community, provided that directives be issued for mutual recognition of diplomas and certificates including those for nurses"[4]. These nursing directives had considerable effect on the education of nurses and midwives and the outcome of the debate within the Committee on Post-Basic Nursing is, at the time of writing, awaited with apprehension. This apprehension may stem from the differences in interpretation of the role of the health visitor/public health nurse in different countries. "The importance of primary care in providing active prevention and promotion activities should likewise never be forgotten"[5].

Most people spend their lives and eventually die in the care of the community nursing services which receive less than 20% of available national resources in the U.K. The difficulties inherent in measuring the benefits of prevention of illness have been used as an excuse for not pursuing research into this field of nursing care. With the acceptance of a definition of 'health' it becomes possible to identify the role of workers who promote 'health' and thus to measure both the absence of 'health' in the lives of individuals and communities and also that state of health which has been promoted.

If similarities in preventive health care can be found in several countries, then the reality of the work will be more creditable. It will not be thought so vulnerable to, for example, directives from the EEC and will also be able to withstand an adverse economic climate. If, indeed, it were possible to prove that a higher standard of health could be attained for a known, lower use of resources, health visiting/public health nursing services might actually thrive in times of financial stress.

It is exceedingly doubtful that the use of the same word 'nurse' means that the 'same nursing service' is provided in each of the European countries. Certainly, the term 'health visitor/public health nurse' does not mean that the same duties are being carried out everywhere. What is important is that nurses have a specific responsibility for the prevention of ill-health and the promotion of good health. 'Health Education' is frequently mentioned as one of the tasks of many of the public health nurses but it is unlikely that there is a common content to this work. Few health visitors in the UK will agree on their job-descriptions and thus it is not surprising that there is considerable variation in the tasks which constitute the work in other countries.

Countries employing public health nurses make frequent reference to 'prevention'. It is to this common factor that critics should attach importance, rather than to the differences in the services operating in the different countries. The similarities are concerned with an emphasis on the importance of the quality of life of the people. This philosophy will manifest itself in policies concerned with the social, economic and environmental aspects of life.

Though there are different points of emphasis and development, in the following examples, they all demonstrate a positive attitude to the promotion of health and prevention of illness.

Denmark

Health Visitors are employed within the National Health Service. In 1978 there were 1,055 health visitors employed by local authorities, giving a ratio of 1:4,800 population[6]. In the work of the health visitor, who has a 10-month post-basic nurse education, emphasis is given to the needs of children with special problems, whether of a health or social nature[7].

France

Nurses, following a 22 month course of training, undertake some preventive health practice in the community - a maternity and child welfare service, a school health service, with a badly-needed home-care service based on particular hospitals being developed in a few areas[8]. There is close relationship between the health and the social welfare systems in which nurses are encouraged to work closely with their colleagues. The decrease in perinatal mortality rates has been taken as an indicator of successful health education.

Germany

The Länder have the main responsibility for the health service but only four of them issue a licence to practice following a twelve-month public health course. Community nursing care is illness-centred and does not yet include prevention or health education[9].

Italy

Quinn describes the basis of the National Health Service as being the promotion of health, prevention of sickness, care and rehabilitation, as well as the improvement of the personal and general environment. She says that by 1975 there were forty-three health health visitor training schools, offering a ten month post-basic nursing course. Health Visitors require authorisation from the Ministry of Labour and Social Security, in addition to that of the Ministry of Health and the Ministry of Education which is needed by all nurses.

Netherlands

Some aspects of public health nursing is offered in the basic three/four years nursing course which is followed by a twenty-two month specialised post-basic public health nurse/health visitor course. "It seems that the Dutch people are perhaps more health concious than us (in the UK). There is a good attendance rate at the child health clinics, and a low infant mortality rate."[10]

Norway

Since 1947, 18,000 health visitors have been educated; there are three post-basic health visitor schools offering a twelve-month course. "In both urban and rural districts the people of Norway demand and expect the services of the health visitors ..... An effort is being made to train other staff to undertake the environmental/sanitary work which presently is being undertaken by the health visitor, so that she will be able to devote more of her time to children."[11]

Poland

The basic nurse education can be followed by a two-year public health nurse course with an emphasis on prophylaxis which is actively continued into practice. Health visitors/public health nurses work in a primary health care team in well patronised health centres.

Health visitors, like other health service professionals, work within the health system of their country. This system reflects the value placed on 'health' by the people of that country. The impetus for the development of the health professionals may be derived from a 'sickness' model of, for example, medicine, or a 'preventive/promotive' model of, for example, education. As stated in 'Formulating Strategies for Health for all by the year 2000', 'health' cannot be achieved by policies in the health sector alone, but nevertheless health staff make a major contribution to this overall plan.

A national strategy guided by ideas of prevention, concerned for the development of constructive rather than destructive health forces, will provide a natural environment in which health visitors/public health nurses can thrive, making their maximum contribution to 'health' in their country. "Since health development both contributes to and results from social and economic development, health policies ideally should form part of overall development policies, thus reflecting the social and economic goals of the government and the people. In this way strategies for the health and social and economic sectors will be mutually supportive, and together contribute to the ultimate goals of the society."[12]

References

1. Moerloose, J de. *Draft Study of Legislation concerning Nursing Services and Education.* Copenhagen: WHO Regional Office for Europe, 1979. p.2.
2. Bridges D.C. *A History of the International Council of Nurses 1899-1964.* London 1967.
3. *Primary Health Care: Report of the International Conference on Primary Health Care, Alma-Alta 1978.* Geneva: WHO 1978.
4. Moerloose, J de. op cit. p.3.
5. *Definition of Parameters of Efficiency in Primary Care and the Role of Nursing in Primary Health Care: Report on two Working Groups, Reykjavik 1975.* Copenhagen: WHO Regional Office for Europe, 1976.
6. Council for the Education and Training of Health Visitors. *Visit to EEC Countries - October 1978.* Hay P. Unpublished Report.
7. Quinn, S. ed. *Nursing in the European Community,* London: Croom Helm. 1980. p.51.
8. Rogers, B.N. et al. *The Study of Social Policy: a Comparative Approach* London: Allen and Unwin, 1979.
9. Quinn, S. op cit. p.74.
10. CETHV. Hay P. op cit.
11. Wilson C.T. *Personal Account of the Health Visitors and the Health Visiting Service in Norway 1978.* North East Polytechnic. Unpublished Report.
12. *Formulating Strategies for Health for all by the year 2000.* Geneva: WHO 1979.

Chapter 9

About the ends and means of Health Visiting

Ruth Schröck

With "An Investigation into the Principles of Health Visiting" (1977)[1] and "The Investigation Debate"[2] (1980), health visitors had made explicit some of the key concepts with which they operate, and had formulated some principles which underlie their practice.

In a conceptual appraisal of their practice, health visitors had attempted to establish a basis for health visiting by

- identifying and clarifying pertinent concepts elucidated from current health visiting practice
- defining health visiting
- relating key concepts in various models to each other and applying these to health visiting practice in order to test their explanatory value and power for that practice
- constructing a conceptual framework of health visiting
- formulating the principles of searching for health needs, stimulating awareness of health needs, influencing health related policy, and facilitating health enhancing activities.

These principles, as they emerged from a thorough examination of what health visitors do or, at any rate, felt that they ought to do, articulated the ideals, aims, purposes or goals of health visiting.

As Clough observed rightly in the "Investigation Debate"[3] "the positive concept of health implies certain objectives and strategies on the part of the health visitor", and one may well take the articulated principles to denote such strategies and objectives. Or, to put it another way, the principles which were formulated in the "Investigation" showed us the ends of health visiting practice.

What health visiting is meant to achieve in the end, some may argue, is

105

perhaps an ideal, and with that they often imply it is unreachable, or that these ends cannot be realized.

I would suggest that the aims, purposes or goals of health visiting may be something that is yet to be achieved, and that we have yet to explain how it is to be realised.

Even if one were to agree that not all the desired ends of health visiting can be achieved by all health visitors all of the time, I would argue that the activities of the health visiting profession as a whole could well demonstrate the achievement of these ends to which individual health visitors may contribute predominantly in one way rather than another, depending on their particular clientele, resources, organisation and specialized knowledge. But even so, the activities of each individual health visitor should and can demonstrably strive towards these ends, even if they are not attainable in an absolute sense by any individual at a particular time and in a particular setting.

The "Debate", and especially Clough's contribution to it,[4] raised two fundamental questions, namely

- is the concept of health (on which the principles of health visiting rest) too global and does it need to be a more specific one to become practically useful?
- what is the relationship of the principles of health visiting to health visiting knowledge?

The concept of health as it was articulated and analyzed in the "Investigation"[5] was felt by many to be so wide that it would be equally useful for all kinds of other people and indeed, that it could be seen to be almost synonymous with other equally global concepts like, for example, education. While I would agree that all such wide concepts need to be re-examined very frequently in order to elicit their functional and, to the purpose in hand, pertinent features, I would not see it to be necessary and, indeed, would consider it to be dangerous to strive for a 'once and for all' settled definition. What is important is that such fundamental concepts as health, education, freedom, democracy and many others which seem to be part of the basic fabric of our society, become personalized and alive in the thinking and understanding of each individual. This demands not only an examination of what they mean to each person but a constant re-examination of what place and power these global ideas have at any given time in our society. Because concepts like health and education and others of a similar kind are so fundamental to everyone's life, I would expect that they should be global rather than restricted or contained. That other people might use them for their own particular ends does not in any case invalidate their use in health visiting or any other enterprise. It seems logical to me that 'health' in its widest sense should be a shared concept which everyone uses. If it is a desirable state of being which nurses and doctors hope that ill people might regain, which health visitors strive to assess, maintain, enhance and protect, which teachers of all kinds tell us about, and which politicians avow to be concerned with, then one must surely hope and expect that they are all talking about the same thing.

I think that the attempt to contain or to concentrate the whole business of health as far as health visitors are concerned is not so much the issue that presents itself by a global concept of health, but that it relates to the question of responsibility. What worries those who feel that the concept of health needs to be more narrowly defined is the assumption of total population care which I think might be implied in the wider expansionist concept of health.

Apart from the question whether some total population care is or should be the responsibility of the health visiting profession, there is the question whether it is in any case possible, and if it is possible, whether it is desirable.

Those who argue that total population health care is not only impossible but undesirable, whether offered by health visitors alone or in cooperation with other caring professions, fear that we would come dangerously near to a paternalistic, if not authoritarian state of affairs.

Another aspect which I think leads to a demand for some sort of restriction or containment of the concept of health is that the more expansionist definitions of health end up with some kind of hope that those who produce this state of health in individuals or in whole populations contribute materially to a state of social well being of those individuals and groups. If the very indefinable state of an individual's or of a population's social well being is then equated with social contentment or happiness, as seems to be implied in some of the more global definitions, then this raises important political and moral questions which health visitors must examine carefully. I cannot, however, see that these questions or debates can or should be avoided by the endeavour to restrict or contain the concept of health. This is not to say that a more focused or a more detailed exposition of what health might mean with specific reference to the ends of health visiting should not be attempted. If this is done with a specific purpose and with some practical application in mind one can envisage a number of useful working definitions which concentrate on or highlight particular features of the more global definitions.

The second question raised by the "Debate"[6] concerned the relationship of the principles of health visiting to health visiting knowledge. Although we now know the value base for health visiting practice, we do not yet know its knowledge base. If we accept that the four principles derived from the value of health and the definition of health visiting constitute the ends of health visiting practice, we need to examine by what means these ends can be achieved. Clearly, knowledge must be part of the means leading to the ends of health visiting practice.

The major question then is how this knowledge can be identified, taught and utilized in the process of health visiting.

In any practice discipline, the search for what is relevant, essential and necessary knowledge must start with a close scrutiny of that practice. The systematic, methodical and goal directed analysis of the concrete behaviour of the practitioners of health visiting must be attempted, if the sometimes remarked upon 'invisibility' of what health visitors define as the focus and the whole reason for their activities is to be remedied. Those who will point to the insubstantial research that already exists about health visitors should examine carefully the difference between research about health visitors and research in health visiting. Sociologists and psychologists who have examined what health visitors do, have done so, rightly, in order to answer sociological or psychological questions. The sociologist may, endeavour to contribute to sociological theory by examining power relationships in a particular group of people, and these may happen to be health visitors. Her investigation must be based on sociological concepts and will be conducted from a sociological perspective. There is no way in which it will explain health visiting in health visiting terms.

Health visiting needs to be examined by health visitors from a health visiting perspective, if one wants to identify health visiting knowledge. This perspective, or conceptual frame-work now exists in the form of the principles of health visiting. What is needed are tools which will allow the health visitor to look, examine, and analyze health visiting practice, and to evaluate it in relation to the stated goals or objectives of health visiting.

A process approach is one way of achieving some part of this analysis. The concrete description of the assessment, planning, implementation, and evaluation of health visiting practice will provide a logical, systematic, and coherent approach to such an investigation. However, it must be remembered that the 'process of health visiting', if one uses the current phrase to describe this examination, is only a tool which can be used effectively or ineffectively. It is not a remedy for all the problems that health visitors may encounter.

The 'process of health visiting' provides a reasoned and logical approach to looking at what actually happens when health visitors engage in their particular activities. It is only one way to explain, to articulate, and to document the work of the health visitor. There are others, and, for example, a systems approach* could be equally useful, or perhaps complementary to the 'process of health visiting' in identifying some of the knowledge utilized in health visiting practice.

Any such approach will indicate some theoretical baselines for health visiting knowledge and its parameters.

Before we can say what knowledge we need from other disciplines, for example, from sociology of psychology, we need to be able to

- articulate key concepts in health visiting practice
- formulate health visiting practice theories
- identify what other disciplines can offer
- select from other disciplines relevant and appropriate knowledge.

The traditional way in which nurses and health visitors constructed their curricula was to start with randomly selected bits of knowledge from a great variety of disciplines largely based on what others thought we needed to know.†

The 'basic' natural and social sciences were taught without any clear idea on the part of anyone what they were to be a basis for. However, it would be unjustified to blame, for example, sociologists for teaching sociology in a way which is entirely appropriate for sociology students although it may be of little relevance or use in that form to health visiting students, if we either do not know what it is that sociologists can offer us, or if we do not tell them what it is of all that they could teach that we really need to learn.

It may be stating the obvious by now to say that the basis of health visiting practice is health visiting knowledge. Selected knowledge derived from a great many disciplines is not basic at all in the sense that it is somehow primary to health visiting knowledge which emerges from it in

* For reference to Systems Approach as in Nursing Concepts of Health Promotion see Chapter 2 The System for Delivery of Health Care. p.29. Zentner J., Murray R. and Levy B.

† The reader is referred to two further discussion documents
1) Time to Learn - Report of the Standing Conference of Representatives of Health Visitor Training Centres, 1979.
2) Report of the Working Party on Curriculum Development, CETHV 1981.

some mysterious fashion, The primary (or basic) knowledge that is of any 'use to the health visitor is that which helps her identify, direct, organise and conduct purposeful activities which are uniquely accomplished in that particular way only by health visitors, that is, she needs primarily health visiting knowledge. Any contributions from other disciplines are only useful, if they can be applied to make these purposeful activities more effective. By being deliberately selected for this purpose from a wide range of available knowledge and by being applied in a particular way within a purposeful activity, this derived knowledge is, as some would say, 'integrated', that is, it becomes part of health visiting knowledge.

There is a dynamic realtionship between the means and ends of health visiting practice which determines what at any time is pertinent health visiting knowledge.

As the principles of health visiting which were formulated in the "Investigation" by those who had been or were practising as health visitors denote the ends of that practice (expressing the value base), so empirical investigations of that practice by, for example, process or systems approaches will identify the means of health visiting practice. these empirical investigations will provide the evidence which in turn can validate the principles originally conceptualised by reliable empirical data (expressing the knowledge base). Principles will emerge which denote more specifically the theoretical (knowledge) base and they in turn will reinforce, modify or change the principles denoting objectives and strategies (or the value base). The conceptual framework will be modified and will change more or less rapidly which in turn will determine empirical investigations from a more or less changed perspective. Further knowledge will emerge and so process will continue. But what is important is that for the first time, this process will lead to an accumulation of health visiting knowledge articulated, documented and used by health visitors from a health visiting perspective. The 'invisible' profession will become 'visible' and, who knows, not only our health care may become increasingly more efffective, but we might even gain in contentment and happiness.

References

1. *An Investigation into the Principles of Health Visiting*, CETHV 1977.
2. *The Investigation Debate*, CETHV 1980
3. Ibid P.15.
4. Ibid P.15.
5. CETHV 1977 Op cit. Chapter 3, P.20.
6. CETHV 1980 Op cit. Chapter 1, P.14.

Contributing Authors

Daman Bahl	SRN, HV Cert., Further Ed. Teachers Cert., HV Tutor, Teachers Cert., FWT Cert., FP Cert. Senior Lecturer, North East London Polytechnic
Sylvia Campbell	SRN, SCM, HV Tutor Cert. Principal Lecturer, Ulster Polytechnic
Phil Connolly	BSc, M.Phil., SRN, HV Tutor Cert. Lecturer in Adult Education (Health Visiting) University of Surrey
Pat Ellis	BSc (Hons), PhD Senior Lecturer, Luton College of Higher Education
Judith Fitton	SRN, SCM, HV Tutor Cert., Dip.Ad.Ed. (Leeds) Lecturer, University of Leeds
Alison McClymont	MSc, SRN, SCM, HV Tutor Cert., Dip.Ad.Ed. Professional Adviser, Council for the Education and Training of Health Visitors
Mary McClymont	SRN, SCM, HV Tutor Cert., BTA Cert., Queens Nurse Principal Lecturer, Stevenage College of Further Education
Ruth Schröck	MA, PhD, DNS (Educ.), SRN, RMN, RNT Senior Lecturer, Dundee College of Technology
Susan Willis	BA (Hons), SRN, SCM, HV Assistant Secretary, Health Visitors' Association
C. Thelma Wilson	BA, FCIS, MISW Principal Lecturer, North East London Polytechnic